Multiple Choice Questions
ENT Head and Neck Surgery
Single Best Answers

Ricardo Abraham Petember Persaud
CCT Otol. (UK), FRCS ORL-HNS (Eng)
MBBS (Lond), MSB (UK), CBiol (UK), DO-HNS, MPhil (Lond), MRCS Gen (Eng),
Consultant ENT, Head Neck and Rhinoplastic Surgeon
Al-Zahra Medical Group
Sharjah and Dubai
PO Box 3499
United Arab Emirates

Emma Jane Gosnell
MBChB MRCS DO-HNS
Trainee Surgeon in Otolaryngology
Fairfield General Hospital
North West Region
United Kingdom

FIRST EDITION 2015

First published 2015 by FAST-PRINT PUBLISHING
Peterborough, England

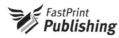

www.fast-print.net/store.php

**Multiple Choice Questions
ENT Head and Neck Surgery
Single Best Answers**

A catalogue record of this book is available from the British Library

ISBN: 978-178456-186-4

An environmentally friendly book printed and bound in England by
www.printondemand-worldwide.com

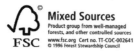

Mixed Sources
Product group from well-managed
forests, and other controlled sources
www.fsc.org Cert no. TT-COC-002641
© 1996 Forest Stewardship Council

PEFC Certified
This product is
from sustainably
managed forests
and controlled
sources
www.pefc.org

This book is made entirely by chain-of-custody materials.

Multiple Choice Questions
ENT Head and Neck Surgery
Single Best Answers

CONTENTS

Acknowledgement

Many thanks to Dr Shahrul Ibrahim for
editing the penultimate manuscript.

1. Which one of the following is inherited as an autosomal dominant condition?

    (a) Cystic fibrosis
    (b) Jervell and Lange-Nielsen
    (c) Treacher Collins
    (d) Alport syndrome
    (e) Usher syndrome

2. Approximately how many mls of saline are needed to make a safe maximum dose of 1% lignocaine without adrenaline for a 70kg man?

    (a) 10
    (b) 20
    (c) 100
    (d) 200
    (e) 400

3. A researcher reports that a new antibiotic is more effective than an established standard for bacterial sinusitis, p = 0.015. Which of the following statement is true?

    (a) The new antibiotic increased relative efficacy by 15%
    (b) The new antibiotic increased absolute efficacy by 15%
    (c) The likelihood of a type 1 error is 1.5%
    (d) The likelihood of a type 11 error is 1.5%
    (e) The likelihood of adequate statistical power is 98.5%

4. A 36-year-old man presents with a hoarse voice, difficulty being heard and is often confused for a woman on the telephone. Videostroboscopy shows a linear depression in the free edge of the true vocal cord. Which of the following is the most likely diagnosis?

   (a) Reinke's oedema
   (b) Singers nodules
   (c) Spasmodic dysphonia
   (d) Sulcus vocalis
   (e) Vocal Cord granuloma

5. Which is the most appropriate therapeutic option for a T2N0M0 glottic carcinoma?

   (a) Radiotherapy
   (b) Chemotherapy
   (c) Surgery and post op radiotherapy
   (d) Chemoradiotherapy
   (e) Primary surgery and modified radical neck dissection

6. A newborn boy presents with a cardiac murmur, ear abnormalities and choanal atresia. Which of the following is the most likely syndrome?

   (a) Alport syndrome
   (b) Pierre-Robin sequence
   (c) CHARGE syndrome
   (d) Cogan's syndrome
   (e) Crouzon syndrome

7. Which test is most suitable to assess the linear analogue scale responses of a group of subjects (n=15) asked to report their perceived pain on 2 consecutive days?

   (a) Pearsons correlation coefficient
   (b) Spearmans rank correlation coefficient
   (c) Two sample (unpaired) Student's t- test
   (d) Two-way analysis of variance (ANOVA)
   (e) Wilcoxon matched pairs test

8. A 45-year-old man presents with acute onset of nausea and vertigo. He is just recovering from infective rhinosinusitis. Examination reveals nystagmus to the left. Which of the following is the most likely diagnosis?

   (a) Labyrinthitis
   (b) Lateral sinus thrombosis
   (c) Meningitis
   (d) Perforation of tympanic membrane
   (e) Subperiosteal abscess

9. With regards to caloric testing, which one of these statements is true?

   (a) Cold water results in nystagmus to the same side
   (b) Cold water results in no nystagmus
   (c) Warm water results in no nystagmus
   (d) Warm water results in nystagmus to the same side
   (e) Warm water results in nystagmus to the opposite side

10. Which congenital deformity typically results in 1.5 turns of the cochlea?

(a) Michel aplasia
(b) Schiebe deformity
(c) Alexander dysplasia
(d) Mondini dysplasia
(e) Enlarged vestibular aqueduct

11. A 3-year-old girl presents with painful left sided swelling in level 2 of the neck associated with otalgia. Ultrasound sound scan reveals the presence of a collection along the left posterior belly of the digastric muscle. Which of the following is the most likely diagnosis?

(a) Bezold's abscess
(b) Citelli's abscess
(c) Extradural abscess
(d) Subdural abscess
(e) Subperiosteal abscess

12. A 28-year-old man presents with a pulsatile swelling in his supraclavicullar fossa. He experiences a cold hand on the same side. Which of the following is the most likely diagnosis?

(a) Branchial cyst
(b) Cervical rib
(c) Sternomastoid tumour
(d) Subclavian artery aneurysm
(e) Glomus jugular tumour

13. Which symptom is not associated with a pharyngeal pouch?

   (a) Halitosis
   (b) Regurgitation
   (c) Weight loss
   (d) Weight gain
   (e) Aspiration pneumonia

14. A 28-year-old amateur singer presents with a 2 month history of a hoarse voice. What is the most likely diagnosis?

   (a) Vocal cord palsy
   (b) Vocal cord nodules
   (c) Vocal cord granuloma
   (d) Squamous cell carcinoma of larynx
   (e) Laryngeal papillomatosis

15. Which of the following is an unusual presentation of a glomus vagale?

   (a) Pulsatile tinnitus
   (b) Recurrent drop attack
   (c) Facial nerve palsy
   (d) Hypoglossal nerve palsy
   (e) Otalgia

16. Where can endolymph be found within the cochlea?

   (a) Scala vestibule
   (b) Scala media
   (c) Scala tympani
   (d) Helicotrema
   (e) Utricle

17. Which artery(s) supply the tonsil?

    (a) Dorsal lingual branches of the lingual artery
    (b) Tonsillar branch of the facial artery
    (c) Ascending pharyngeal artery from external carotid
    (d) Descending palatine branch of maxillary artery
    (e) All of the above

18. A 60-year-old man presents with unilateral hearing loss and tinnitus. Pure tone audiometry reveals asymmetrical sensori-neural hearing loss. A MR scan of the CPA/IAM was subsequently organised and the neuro-radiologist reported a lesion with a broad base and bilateral dural tails in the cerebellar pontine angle. What is the most likely diagnosis?

    (a) Meningioma
    (b) Acoustic neuroma
    (c) Vestibular schwannoma
    (d) Cholesteatoma
    (e) Cholesteral granuloma

19. A 65-year-old man presents with dry mouth and dental caries. He takes omeprazole daily for the last 2 years. What is the single most likely diagnosis?

    (a) Geographic tongue
    (b) Erythroplakia
    (c) Mucocoeles
    (d) Sjogrens
    (e) Xerostomia

20. A 25-year-old man presents with suspicion of otitis media with effusion. Tympanometry reveals peak compliance of -180daPa. What is the single most likely tympanogram?

   (a) Type As
   (b) Type Ad
   (c) Type B
   (d) Type C1
   (e) Type C2

21. What is the risk of malignant transformation in a patient with oral lichen planus for over 10 years?

   (a) 0%
   (b) 5%
   (c) 10%
   (d) 50%
   (e) 100%

22. A 65-year-old male farmer presents with a bleeding lesion on the upper part of the pinna. Examination reveals a 1 cm ulcerative lesion with heaped up edges and a palpable level II lymph node. Which of the following is the most likely diagnosis?

   (a) Basal cell carcinoma
   (b) Keratoacanthoma
   (c) Gouty tophi
   (d) Squamous cell carcinoma
   (e) Pinna cellulitis

23. A 39-year-old patient presents with suspected non-organic hearing loss. Which of the following is the most appropriate OPD diagnostic test?

   (a) Free field testing
   (b) Pure tone audiogram
   (c) Stenger's test
   (d) Distraction testing
   (e) Conditioned response audiometry

24. What is the most likely corresponding eponymous name for a multinucleated cell found in granulomatous conditions?

   (a) Kupffer cells
   (b) Langerhans cells
   (c) Langhan cells
   (d) Michaels's bodies
   (e) Mikulicz's cells

25. A 38-year-old man presents with normal symmetry and tone at rest but no forehead movement and incomplete eye closure. What is the House-Brackman (HB) grading of facial nerve palsy?

   (a) HB Grade II
   (b) HB Grade III
   (c) HB Grade IV
   (d) HB Grade V
   (e) HB Grade VI

26. A 45-year-old Chinese woman presents with epistaxis. Examination and biopsy reveals a nasopharyngeal carcinoma confined to the nasopharynx with no palpable neck nodes. What is the TNM staging?

   (a) T1N0M0
   (b) T1N1M0
   (c) T2N0M0
   (d) T3N1M0
   (e) T4N0M0

27. A 25-year-old male motorcyclist presents with a left facial nerve palsy following an accident that involved him landing on the back of his head. He also has bleeding from his left ear and right beating nystagmus associated with ipsilateral profound hearing loss. What is the most likely diagnosis?

   (a) Transverse temporal bone fracture
   (b) Facial nerve neuroma
   (c) Facial nerve transection
   (d) Bell's palsy
   (e) Moebius syndrome

28. A 25-year-old male surfer presents with recurrent otitis externa and conductive hearing loss. Exam shows bilateral sessile masses adjacent to tympanic membrane in the external auditory canal. What is the most likely diagnosis?

   (a) Pyogenic granuloma
   (b) Exostoses
   (c) Osteoma
   (d) Ear canal polyp
   (e) Furunclosis

29. A 27-year-old man presents with intermittent facial nerve palsy and a swollen fissured tongue. Which of the following is the most likely diagnosis?

(a) Guillain Barre syndrome
(b) Lyme disease
(c) Maffucci syndrome
(d) Melkersson-Rosenthal syndrome
(e) Syphilis

30. A 48-year-old caucasian man presents with an irregular lesion on the back of his neck that has enlarged and started bleeding. The lesion is has a variegated appearance. What is the most likely diagnosis?

(a) Acral lentiginous melanoma
(b) Basal cell carcinoma
(c) Benign naevus
(d) Superficial spreading malignant melanoma
(e) Squamous cell carcinoma

31. A 17-year-old girl presents to accident and emergency having taken an overdose. She complains of severe tinnitus. Which of the following drugs is most likely to be responsible?

(a) Aspirin
(b) Propranolol
(c) Phenytoin
(d) Rosperidone
(e) Frusemide

32. A 35-year-old man presents with an injury to his neck that is associated with hoarseness and stridor. Which of the following is the single most likely injury?

   (a) Temporal bone fracture
   (b) Cerebrospinal fluid leak
   (c) Mandibular fracture
   (d) Laryngotracheal injury
   (e) Oesophageal perforation

33. A 64-year-old man presents with a tumour of the larynx, which extends into the subglottis. Examination reveals a single unilateral node that is about 1.5 cm in size. No metastases are evident on CT/MRI.   What is the TNM stage?

   (a) T1N1M0
   (b) T2N0M1
   (c) T2N1M0
   (d) T2N0M0
   (e) T3N1M0

34. A 78-year-old woman presents with tinnitus, headache, jaw claudication and diplopia. Her blood test reveals a raised ESR. What is the most likely diagnosis?

   (a) Herpes zoster
   (b) Ramsay Hunt syndrome
   (c) Sinusitis
   (d) Temporal arteritis
   (e) Trigeminal neuralgia

35. A 3-month-old boy presents with gradually worsening noisy breathing that is especially noticeable when he eats or is supine. He is on a lower centile for weight gain and has poor food intake. What is the likely diagnosis?

   (a) Choanal atresia
   (b) Laryngeal papillomatosis
   (c) Laryngomalacia
   (d) Piriform aperture stenosis
   (e) Vocal cord palsy

36. A 28-year-old woman presents with intermittent severe temporofacial pain. Each episode begins with severe pain in and around the right ear radiating across the right side of the face and down to the right jaw. More recently she describes severe pain when touching her lower lip on the right. Her clinical and neurological examination is normal apart from observing an internuclear ophthalmoplegia. What is the most likely diagnosis?

   (a) Temporal arteritis
   (b) Sphenopalatine ganglion neuralgia
   (c) Multiple Sclerosis
   (d) Motor neurone disease
   (e) Trigeminal neuralgia

37. A 4-year-old boy presents with hearing loss. Examination reveals mandibular and midfacial hypoplasia along with down slanting palpabre fissures. What is the most likely syndrome in this case?

   (a) Pendred
   (b) CHARGE
   (c) Sticklers
   (d) Treacher-Collins
   (e) Turners

38. A 10-year-old girl presents with red spots on the buccal mucosa, conjunctivitis, otitis media, rhinitis and maculopapular rash. Which is the most likely infectious disease?

    (a) Chicken-pox
    (b) Mumps
    (c) Measles
    (d) Scarlet fever
    (e) Hand, foot & mouth disease

39. A 54-year-old man presents with several months of a foul smelling discharge from his right ear. The discharge prevents him from going out with his friends. Otoscopy reveals an attic perforation combined with a dark brown wax-like material. What is the most likely diagnosis?

    (a) Otitis externa
    (b) Chronic serous otitis media
    (c) Cholesteatoma
    (d) Otospongiosis
    (e) Otosyphilis

40. A 70-year-old man presents with an intermittent vertigo which began 2 months ago after a minor head injury. He described attacks lasting for 1–2 minutes usually when turning over to the right side in bed. What is the most likely diagnosis?

    (a) Migraine
    (b) BPPV
    (c) Menieres disease
    (d) Acute labyrinthitis
    (e) Vertebro-basilar ischaemia

41. A 68 year old gentleman presents to clinic with a 0.4 cm septal perforation. Which symptom is more often associated with a small septal perforation?

    (a) Epistaxis
    (b) Crusting
    (c) Rhinorrhoea
    (d) Whistling
    (e) Difficulty with breathing

42. A 39-year-old woman presents complains of a 2-year history of intermittent sore red eyes, bilateral hearing loss, tinnitus and difficulty discriminating sounds in background noise. Otoscopic examination is normal. Pure tone audiogram reveals bilateral hearing loss at 2 kHz and a speech audiogram showed optimal discrimination score of 80 percent. What is the most likely diagnosis?

    (a) Cogan's syndrome
    (b) Wegener's granulomatosis
    (c) Syphilis
    (d) Polyarteritis nodosa
    (e) Sjögren's syndrome

43. A 50-year-old male patient presents with chronic rhinosinusitis. Recently, he complained of bloody nasal discharge, cough and shortness of breath. The chest X ray shows a diffuse area of consolidation and cavities in the multiple lobes of the lungs. Urinalysis shows red blood cells cast and protein. What is the most likely diagnosis?

    (a) Wegener's
    (b) Sarcoidosis
    (c) Pneumonia
    (d) Carcinoma of the bronchus
    (e) Tuberculosis

44. Which area of the upper airway is usually involved in sarcoidosis?

   (a) Supraglottis
   (b) Glottis
   (c) Subglottis
   (d) Trachea
   (e) Saccule

45. During cold steel tonsillectomy, which is the most appropriate instrument to dissect the tonsil from its underlying attachments?

   (a) Freer's elevator
   (b) Gwynne Evans dissector
   (c) Mollison's pillar retractor
   (d) St Claire Currette
   (e) Boyle's-Davis

46. A 29-year-old childless male presents complaining of recurrent rhinosinusitis. Investigations reveals obstructive azoospermia and bronchiectasis but normal ciliary motility. In this case, which of the following syndromes is most likely?

   (a) CHARGE syndrome
   (b) Kartagener's syndrome
   (c) Osler-Weber-Rendu syndrome
   (d) Pierre Robin syndrome
   (e) Young's syndrome

47. Hereditary haemorrhagic telangectasia (HHT) is a condition diagnosed on the presence of four criteria, known as "curacao criteria". Which is not one of the criteria?

(a) Multiple telangiectasia
(b) Recurrent epistaxis
(c) First-degree family member with HHT
(d) Abnormal clotting
(e) Visceral arteriovenous malformations

48. Which sinus does not drain into the hiatus semilunaris?

(a) Maxillary sinus
(b) Frontal sinus
(c) Anterior ethmoidal sinus
(d) Posterior ethmoidal sinus
(e) None of the above

49. A 58-year-old man presents with difficulty breathing through his nose because of a long standing bulbous lesion on his nose which has become ruddy and vascular in appearance. What is the most likely diagnosis?

(a) Basal cell carcinoma
(b) Squamous cell carcinoma
(c) Rhinophyma
(d) Papilloma
(e) Haemangioma

50. The following statements are true of angioedema, EXCEPT:

(a) The potent vasodilator, bradykinin plays a critical role angioedema and therefore the condition may be a side effect of ACE inhibitors such as enalopril
(b) Hereditary angioedema exhibits an autosomal dominant pattern of inheritance
(c) Acute treatment of hereditary angioedema includes anti-histamine, steroids and/or adrenaline.
(d) Angioedema may be due to an autosomal disorder involving antibody formation against C1 esterase inhibitor.
(e) Consumption of NSAIDs or vasodilator foods such as alcohol or cinnamon can increase the probability of an angioedema episode in susceptible patients.

51. A 3-year-old girl presents with history of upper respiratory tract infection and a red swollen eye. There is no proptosis or chemosis and vision is normal. What is the most likely diagnosis?

(a) Preseptal cellulitis
(b) Orbital cellulitis
(c) Pott's puffy tumour
(d) Cavernous sinus thrombosis
(e) Cerebral abscess

52. Which of these diseases is Epstein Barr Virus not associated with?

(a) Infectious mononucleosis
(b) Nasopharyngeal carcinoma
(c) Hairy cell leukaemia
(d) Burkitt's lymphoma
(e) T-cell lymphoma

53. What surgical instrument is used to reinsert a displaced tracheostomy tube?

   (a) Travers retractor
   (b) Jolls retractor
   (c) Negus laryngoscope
   (d) Tilley Henkel foceps
   (e) Trousseau tracheal dilator

54. A 37-year-old woman presents with pyrexia of unknown origin in association with a diffuse painless   right sided parotid swelling, right facial nerve palsy, hilar lymphadenopathy and nasal crusting with streaks of blood in nasal mucus. What is the single most appropriate investigation?

   (a) ACE
   (b) Blood glucose
   (c) MPO
   (d) RAST
   (e) Thyroid function tests

55. The structures of the lateral face and neck are formed from paired branchial arches, pouches and clefts. Which pouch/ pouches contribute to the parathyroid glands?

   (a) first and second
   (b) second and third
   (c) third and fourth
   (d) fourth and fifth
   (e) fifth and sixth

56. Which is the most likely causative virus for Aseptic meningitis?

    (a) Coxsackie virus
    (b) Parvovirus
    (c) Rotavirus
    (d) Adenovirus
    (e) Astrovirus

57. Through which skull base foramen does the mandibular division of the trigeminal nerve pass?

    (a) Superior orbital fissure
    (b) Foramen rotundum
    (c) Foramen ovale
    (d) Foramen spinosum
    (e) Foramen lacerum

58. A 65-year-old African man presents with a large, smooth goitre. He says it has been enlarging for at least 15 years. What is the most appropriate pathology?

    (a) De Quervain's thyroiditis
    (b) Endemic goitre
    (c) Follicular adenoma
    (d) Riedel's thyroiditis
    (e) Hashimoto's disease

59. With regards to measures of central tendency in statistics, which of the following statements is true?

(a) The mean is always a good measure of central tendency
(b) The mode is the sum of all the variables divided by the number of variables
(c) There is only one mode in any given distribution
(d) The median is not the middle of the distribution
(e) The mean, mode and median are equal in normal distributions

60. From how many pharyngeal arches does the tongue develop?

(a) One
(b) Two
(c) Three
(d) Four
(e) Five

61. To compare the systolic BP measurements of four independent groups (n=80)/group of subjects. What is the single most suitable statistical test?

(a) two sample (unpaired) Students t-test
(b) two way analysis of variance (ANOVA)
(c) Wilcoxon matched pair test
(d) One way analysis of variance
(e) Mann-Whitney U Test

62. The point on the skull corresponding to the posterior end of the parietomastoid suture is known as...

    (a) Asterion
    (b) Bregma
    (c) Inion
    (d) Rhinion
    (e) Pterion

63. What diagnostic blood test is more important for hereditary angio-oedema?

    (a) C1 esterase inhibitor level
    (b) Erythrocyte Sedimentation Ratio
    (c) Antinuclear antibody
    (d) Anti-neutrophil cytoplasmic antibody
    (e) Angiotensin-Converting Enzyme level

64. Which of the following is not a branch of the facial nerve?

    (a) Temporal nerve
    (b) Posterior auricular nerve
    (c) Lesser superficial petrosal nerve
    (d) Chorda tympani nerve
    (e) Nerve to stapedius muscle

65. A 37 year old man presents with dysphagia and subsequently achalasia is diagnosed. Which one of the following features is present in achalasia?

(a) Fibrosis associated with a least moderate oesophagitis
(b) Lack of sensitivity of the lower oesophageal sphincter to gastrin
(c) Loss of ganglion cells in Auerbach's plexus
(d) Low pressures within the lower oesophageal sphincter
(e) Vigorous peristalsis in the body of the oesophagus

66. A 60 degree Z-plasty results in lengthening of the scar by how much percent?

(a) 15
(b) 25
(c) 50
(d) 75
(e) 100

67. The following statements on clinical trials and evidence-based medicine is correct?

    (a) Treatments supported by a single RCT are said to have level 1a evidence
    (b) An intention to treat analysis means that patients outcomes are analysed according to the treatment that they received, as opposed to the group to which they were randomised
    (c) A study has a type II error if it finds an effect or difference when none exists
    (d) An absolute risk reduction (ARR) is the risk in the control group minus the risk in the treated group, and is the inverse of the number needed to treat (NNT)
    (e) A p-value of less that 0.05 means that the probability of a result occurring by chance is less than 1 in 5.

68. A 39-year-old woman presents complaining of her scapula protruding when she pushes open a door 4 weeks after a neck dissection. Which nerve has most likely been damaged?

    (a) C5
    (b) C6
    (c) C7
    (d) C5-C7
    (e) C8

69. Following a wisdom tooth extraction, a 35-year-old male complains of loss of taste on the left side of his tongue and severe bleeding from the left side of his tongue which he has bitten. What is the most likely nerve to be involved?

(a) Hypoglossal nerve
(b) Glossopharyngeal nerve
(c) Lingual nerve
(d) Anterior palatine nerve
(e) Cervical sympathetic plexus

70. Damage to the external laryngeal nerve causes which one of the following?

(a) Lengthening of the vocal cord
(b) Abduction of the vocal cord
(c) Adduction of the vocal cord
(d) Shortening of the vocal cord
(e) No change in the vocal cord

71. Which of the following drugs can be used to treat excessive sneezing associated with allergic rhinosinusitis?

(a) Azelastine
(b) Ipratropium bromide
(c) Montelukast
(d) Prolonged courses of systemic corticosteroids
(e) Sodium cromoglycate

72. What is the recommended diagnostic investigation for salivary calculi?

(a) Bimanual palpation
(b) Ultrasound scan
(c) X-ray
(d) Sialogram
(e) MRI scan

73. A 56 year old man presents with a genuine sudden sensori-neural hearing loss in one ear and normal hearing in the other ear. Which of the following tuning fork test results are correct?

(a) AC > BC both ears, Weber lateralizes to the right ear
(b) AC >BC right ear, BC >AC left ear, Weber lateralizes to the right ear
(c) AC > BC left ear, BC>AC right ear, Weber lateralizes to the right ear
(d) AC > BC left ear, Webers lateralizes to the left ear
(e) AC > BC right ear, BC >AC left ear, Webers lateralizes to the left

74. Which cranial nerve sends secretomotor fibres to the parotid gland?

(a) Vagus nerve
(b) Glossopharyngeal nerve
(c) Facial nerve
(d) Trigeminal nerve
(e) Hypoglossal nerve

75. Which fo the following topical aural preparation contains clotrimazole?

  (a) Ofloxacin
  (b) Gentisone
  (c) Canestan
  (d) Betnovate
  (e) Synalar ointment

76. A 60-year-old male worker presents with a blood nasal stained discharge from his nose. He works in a nickel factory. Which is the most likely diagnosis?

  (a) Adenocarcinoma
  (b) Adenoid cystic carcinoma
  (c) Inverted papilloma
  (d) Squamous cell carcinoma
  (e) Benign nasal polyps

77. A 49-year-old male taxi driver presents complaining of snoring. He has had three car accidents and suffers from claustrophobia. His body mass index is normal. A sleep study confirms moderate obstructive sleep apnoea. What would be the most appropriate management option?

  (a) Weight loss
  (b) Exercise
  (c) Oxygen therapy
  (d) Mandibular advancement splint
  (e) Uvuloplasty

78. Which of the following steroids has the greatest glucocorticoid effect?

    (a) Hydrocortisone
    (b) Triamcinolone
    (c) Methyprednisolone
    (d) Betamethasone
    (e) Deflazacort

79. With regards to oncological staging, which stage of disease is given to a patient with T1N1MO laryngeal carcinoma?

    (a) I
    (b) II
    (c) III
    (d) IV
    (e) V

80. A 25-year-old male professional surfer presents with recurrent otitis externa and moderate conductive hearing loss. Examination reveals bilateral sessile masses adjacent to tympanic membrane in the external auditory canal. What is the most appropriate initial hearing device?

    (a) In-the-canal (ITC) hearing aid
    (b) Bone conduction hearing aid
    (c) Bone anchored hearing aid
    (d) Vented behind-the-ear (BTE) hearing aid
    (e) Cochlear implant

81. A 39-year-old man presents with a parotid gland mass. The surgeon would like to know if the lesion extends to the deep lobe of the parotid gland. Which of the following is the most appropriate imaging modality?

    (a) Ultrasound
    (b) CT scan with contrast
    (c) Gadolinium enhanced MRI scan
    (d) MRI STIR sequence
    (e) MRI non echo planar diffusion weighted

82. A 12-year-old Down child presents with otitis media with effusion proven over multiple time points, resulting in reduced hearing. What is the most appropriate management?

    (a) Repeat hearing test with 6 week time interval
    (b) Repeat hearing test in 3 months
    (c) Recommend hearing aids
    (d) Insert grommets
    (e) Insert grommets and adenoidectomy

83. A 45-year-old man presents with a 4-month history of persistent ear ache and some discomfort swallowing but no weight loss. He drinks 10 units of alcohol each day for the last 5 years. Examination reveals a 3 cm cancerous ulcer in the left piriform fossa extending from the medial wall to the lateral wall. The vocal folds were mobile and symmetrical. Neck examination was normal. What is the TNM stage?

    (a) T1N0M0
    (b) T1N1M0
    (c) T1N1aM0
    (d) T1N1bM0
    (e) T2N0M0

84. Congenital cholesteatoma formation involves the persistence of a small nest of stratified squamous epithelial cells within the middle ear. This is based on which theory?

   (a) Acquired inclusion
   (b) Amniotic fluid contamination
   (c) Squamous metaplasia
   (d) Epidermoid formation
   (e) Epithelial migration

85. With regards of middle ear anatomy, which structure lies lateral to the saccule?

   (a) Lateral semi-circular canal
   (b) Promontory
   (c) Sinus tympani
   (d) Oval window
   (e) Round window

86. If a canal wall down procedure is used to treat a postero-superior mesotympanic cholesteatoma, where would be the most likely site of residual disease?

   (a) facial recess
   (b) mesotympanic
   (c) hypotympanic
   (d) sinus tympani
   (e) Eustachian tube

87. Which bacteria are commonly associated with malignant otitis externa?

   (a) Staphylococcus spp.
   (b) Streptococcus spp.
   (c) Pseudomonas aeruginosa
   (d) Moraxella catarrhalis
   (e) Candida albicans

88. A 32-year-old female presents with tinnitus that is exacerbated by external noise. Examination shows objective tinnitus. Review of the tympanic membrane shows movement in synchrony to the tinnitus. What is the most likely diagnosis?

   (a) Stapedius myoclonus
   (b) Tensor tympani myoclonus
   (c) Palatal myoclonus
   (d) Glomus tympanicum
   (e) Spontaneous otoacoustic emissions

89. How much cocaine is present in 5mls of Moffett's solution containing 2mls of 10% cocaine?

   (a) 200mcg
   (b) 200mg
   (c) 100mg
   (d) 20mg
   (e) 10mg

90. A 45-year-old Thai man presents with rhinorrhoea and foul smelling discharge from his nose. He wife says that his nose has been growing. He also has some nodules on his hands. What is the most likely infective organism?

(a) Actinomyces
(b) Rochalimaea (Bartonella) henselae
(c) Rhinosporidium seeberi
(d) Bacteroides spp
(e) Klebsiella rhinoscleromatis

91. Pleomorphic adenoma within the parotid gland carries a small risk of malignant transformation – what percentage is routinely quoted?

(a) 1% for every one year
(b) 5% for every one year
(c) 10% for every one year
(d) 2% if <5 years, 10% if over 15 years
(e) 5% if <5 years, 15% if over 15 years

92. A 49-year-old man presents complaining of asymmetrical tonsils. On examination he was found to have a medially displaced right tonsil. A CT scan report stated that he had a solid lesion in the pre-styloid compartment of his parapharyngeal space. What is the most likely diagnosis?

(a) Metastatic lesion
(b) Salivary gland lesion
(c) Neurogenic lesion
(d) Lymphoma
(e) Primary tonsillar lesion

93. A 64-year-old man presents with a history of bilateral nasal blockage. He has derived temporary relief with an 'over-the-counter' decongestant from the pharmacy he has been using consistently for 3 months. What is the most likely diagnosis?

    (a) Rhinitis medicamentosa
    (b) Atrophic rhinitis
    (c) Perennial allergic rhinitis
    (d) Wegener's granulomatosis
    (e) Nasal polyps

94. A 20-year-old man presents complaining of a persistent right-sided nasal obstruction. He underwent a manipulation under anaesthetic 10 days after nasal trauma. What is the most likely diagnosis?

    (a) Deviation nasal bones
    (b) Deviated nasal septum
    (c) Foreign body
    (d) Removal of inferior turbinates
    (e) Rhinolith

95. What is the most appropriate genetic description for a normal gene involved in the regulation of cell growth?

    (a) Oncogene
    (b) Proto-oncogene
    (c) Tumour suppressor gene
    (d) Allele
    (e) Wild type

96. A 14-year-old boy presents with conductive hearing loss, with significant whitish discolouration of the tympanic membrane surrounding a healed monomeric segment of the drum. The patient previously had 2 sets of grommets. Which of the following is the most appropriate diagnosis?

   (a) Cochlear otosclerosis
   (b) Cogan's syndrome
   (c) Refsum's syndrome
   (d) Usher's syndrome
   (e) Tympanosclerosis

97. Which of the following statements is TRUE of meiosis?

   (a) All the resulting cells have the same genetic material
   (b) The daughter cells have the same genetic material as the mother cell
   (c) The process occurs in all cells
   (d) It is a fundamental process in germ cell
   (e) Is the same as mitosis

98. A 67-year-old woman presents with hearing loss on the left and a decreased sensation along the floor of the ear canal and conchal bowl in comparison to the right side. Which is the single most likely eponymous name?

   (a) Hitselberger's
   (b) Hennebert
   (c) Furstenberg
   (d) Tullio phenomenon
   (e) Holman-Miller

99. A 52-year-old woman presents with a gradual hearing loss showing a moderate slope towards the high frequencies but disproportionately severe decrease in speech discrimination. What is the single most likely diagnosis?

(a) Cogan's syndrome
(b) Inner ear condudive presbyacusis
(c) Neural presbyacusis
(d) Sensory presbyacusis
(e) Strial presbyacusis

100. Which of the following pathological lesion is divided histologically into 3 grades: low, intermediate and high?

(a) Adenocarcinoma
(b) Pleomorphic adenoma
(c) Adenoid cystic carcinoma
(d) Mucoepidermoid carcinoma
(e) Salivary mucocele

101. Which of the following nerves supply the skin over the mastoid:

(a) Vagus
(b) Facial
(c) Trigeminal
(d) Greater auricular
(e) Spinal accessory

102. A 70 year old sheep farmer presents with increasing cluminess, poor concentration and heightened sense of smell. What is the most likely explanation for his symptoms?

   (a) ORF infection
   (b) Shy-Drager syndrome
   (c) Brucellosis
   (d) Organophosphate poisoning
   (e) Alzheimer's disease
   (f)

103. Human papilloma virus is associated with an increase in cancer mainly in which anatomical area?

   (a) Tongue base
   (b) Tonsils
   (c) pharynx
   (d) lateral tongue
   (e) Larynx

104. A 55-year-old male farmer presents with a lesion on his under the angle of the mandible that grows rapidly and then regresses. What is the most likely diagnosis?

   (a) Benign naevus
   (b) Squamous cell carcinoma
   (c) Keratoacanthoma
   (d) Papilloma
   (e) Sebaceous cyst

105. Which nerves are involved in the oral phase of swallowing?

   (a) Trigeminal and vagus
   (b) Facial and vagus
   (c) Glossopharyngeal and vagus
   (d) Trigeminal and facial
   (e) Trigeminal and glossopharyngeal

106. A 10-year-old girl presents with fever, conjunctivitis, fissuring of the lips, strawberry tongue, swelling of the extremities, cervical lymphadenopathy and peripheral desquamation of the palms and soles of the feet. Which is the most likely infectious disease?

   (a) Hand, foot & mouth disease
   (b) Lyme disease
   (c) Steven-Johnson syndrome
   (d) Scarlet fever
   (e) Kawasaki disease

107. Sarcoidosis is an example of which type of hypersensitivity reaction?

   (a) Type I
   (b) Type II
   (c) Type III
   (d) Type IV
   (e) Type V

108. A 18-year-old female rugby player presents with a positive monospot test and a palpable mass below the costal margin on the left hand side of the abdomen. What would you advise her?

   (a)   Change contraceptive pill
   (b)   Do not immerse in water
   (c)   Avoid contact sports
   (d)   Stop drinking alcohol
   (e)   Stop smoking

109. During a full face lift, which nerve is considered to be most at risk of damage?

   (a)   The auriculotemporal nerve
   (b)   The buccal branch of the facial nerve
   (c)   The frontal branch of the facial nerve
   (d)   The great auricular nerve
   (e)   The marginal mandibular branch of the facial nerve

110. A 69-year-old male hard wood worker presents with a blood-stained nasal. Which is the most likely diagnosis?

   (a)   Adenocarcinoma
   (b)   Adenoid cystic carcinoma
   (c)   Inverted papilloma
   (d)   Squamous cell carcinoma
   (e)   Benign nasal polyps

111. Which is the most appropriate dynamic test to assess pulmonary function in asthmatic patients?

    (a) Nasal inspiratory peak flow
    (b) Nasal expiratory peak flow
    (c) Peak flow
    (d) Rhinostereometry
    (e) Spirometry

112. What is the most appropriate investigation for diagnosing cervical cystic hygroma in a child?

    (a) USS
    (b) FNAC
    (c) MRI
    (d) CT
    (e) MRA

		PAPER ONE
		Answers
1.	C	Treacher Collins
2.	B	20mls *(max safe dose for lignocaine without adrenaline 3mg/kg)*
3.	C	The likelihood of a type 1 error is 1.5%
4.	D	Sulcus vocalis
5.	A	Radiotherapy
6.	C	CHARGE syndrome
7.	E	Wilcoxon matched pairs test
8.	A	Labyrinthitis
9.	D	Warm water results in nystagmus to the same side *(COWS- cold opposite, warm same)*
10.	D	Mondini dysplasia
11.	B	Citelli's abscess
12.	D	Subclavian artery aneurysm
13.	D	Weight gain
14.	B	Vocal cord nodules
15.	C	Facial nerve palsy
16.	B	Scala media
17.	A	All of the above
18.	A	Meningioma
19.	E	Xerostomia
20.	E	Type C2
21.	B	5%
22.	D	Squamous cell carcinoma
23.	C	Stenger's test
24.	B	C Langhan cells
25.	C	HB grade IV
26.	A	T1N1M0
27.	A	Transverse temporal bone fracture
28.	B	Exostoses
29.	D	Melkersson-Rosenthal syndrome
30.	D	Superficial spreading malignant melanoma

31.	A	Aspirin
32.	D	Laryngotracheal injury
33.	C	T2N1M0
34.	D	Temporal arteritis
35.	C	Laryngomalacia
36.	C	Multiple sclerosis
37.	D	Treacher-collins
38.	C	Measles
39.	C	Cholesteatoma
40.	B	BPPV
41.	D	Whistling
42.	A	Cogan's syndrome
43.	A	Wegener's
44.	A	Supraglottis
45.	B	Gwynne Evans dissector
46.	E	Young's syndrome
47.	D	Abnormal clotting
48.	D	Posterior ethmoidal sinus
49.	C	Rhinophyma
50.	C	Acute treatment of hereditary angioedema includes anti-histamine, steroids and/or adrenaline *(requires FFP or C1 esterase inhibitor preparation)*.
51.	A	Preseptal cellulitis
52.	C	Hairy cell leukaemia *(EBV is associated with oral hairy cell leukoplakia)*
53.	E	Trousseau tracheal dilator
54.	A	ACE
55.	C	Third and fourth
56.	A	Coxsackie virus
57.	C	Foramen ovale *(mnemonic: MALE-mandibular division of the trigeminal nerve, accessory meningeal artery, lesser petrosal nerve and emissary vein)*
58.	B	Endemic goitre
59.	E	The mean, mode and median are equal in

		normal distributions
60.	D	Four
61.	D	One way analysis of variance
62.	A	Asterion
63.	A	C1 esterase inhibitor level
64.	C	Lesser superficial petrosal nerve
65.	C	Loss of ganglion cells in Auerbach's plexus
66.	D	75
67.	D	An absolute risk reduction (ARR) is the risk in the control group minus the risk in the treated group, and is the inverse of the number needed to treat (NNT)
68.	D	C5-7 *(long thoracic nerve of Bell)*
69.	C	Lingual nerve
70.	E	No change in the vocal cord
71.	A	Azelastine
72. x3	B	AC >BC right ear, BC >AC left ear, Weber lateralizes to the right ear
73.	A	Iodoform, benzoin & storax
74.	B	Glossopharyngeal nerve
75.	C	Canestan
76.	D	Squamous cell carcinoma
77.	D	Mandibular advancement splint
78.	D	Betamethasone
79.	C	III
80.	B	Bone conduction hearing aid
81.	D	MRI STIR sequence
82.	C	Recommend hearing aids
83.	C	T1N1aM0
84.	D	Epidermoid formation theory
85.	D	Gadolinium
86.	D	Oval window
87.	C	Pseudomonas aeruginosa
88.	B	Tensor tympani myoclonus
89.	B	200mg
90.	C	Rhinosporidium seeberi

91.	D	2% if <5 years, 10% if over 15 years
92.	B	Salivary gland lesion
93.	A	Rhinitis medicamentosa
94.	B	Deviated nasal septum
95.	C	Tumour suppressor gene
96.	E	Tympanosclerosis
97.	D	It is a fundamental process in germ cell
98.	A	Hitselberger's
99.	C	Neural presbyacusis
100.	D	Mucoepidermoid carcinoma
101.	D	Greater auricular nerve
102.	D	Organophosphate poisoning (also known as Sheep dip)
103.	B	Tonsils (followed by tongue base)
104.	C	Keratoacanthoma
105.	D	Trigeminal and Facial
106.	E	Kawasaki
107.	D	Type IV hypersensitivity reaction
108.	C	Avoid contact sports
109.	C	The frontal branch of the facial nerve
110.	A	Adenocarcinoma
111.	C	Peak flow
112.	C	MRI

1. Which of the following conditions is not associated with anosmia?

    (a) Kallmann syndrome
    (b) Parkinson's disease
    (c) Alzheimer's disease
    (d) Zinc deficiency
    (e) Down syndrome

2. An ENT Surgeon wants to determine whether a history of childhood tonsillectomy affects rates of adult atopic disease. He assembles a group of adults with and without atopic disease and then compares the rates of tonsillectomy by reviewing their records. This is an example of which type of study?

    (a) Prospective observational study
    (b) Retrospective observational study
    (c) Case-control study
    (d) Case- series study
    (e) Randomised controlled study

3. A 54-year-old woman presents with a tumour confined to a mobile left vocal cord but no palpable cervical nodes. What is the TNM stage?

    (a) T1N0M0
    (b) T1N1M0
    (c) T1N1M1
    (d) T2N0M0
    (e) T2N1M0

4. A 70-year old man presents with sabre-shaped tibia and a unilateral facial nerve palsy. Which of the following is the most likely diagnosis?

    (a) Leprosy
    (b) Lyme disease
    (c) Parotid tumour
    (d) Squamous cell carcinoma
    (e) Syphilis

5. Following right tympanomastoid surgery for a cholesteatoma complicated a fistula in the lateral semicircular canal, the patient wakes up feeling extremely dizzy. A Weber tuning fork test goes to the left suggesting a right dead ear. What is the most likely type of nystagmus to be present?

    (a) Bidirectional
    (b) Downbeat
    (c) Horizontal to the left
    (d) Horizontal to the right
    (e) No nystagmus

6. In which of the following congenital deformity is a cochlear implant contraindicated?

    (a) Michel aplasia
    (b) Schiebe deformity
    (c) Alexander dysplasia
    (d) Mondini dysplasia
    (e) Enlarged vestibular aqueduct

7.   A 63-year-old woman presents with fever, drowsiness, lethargy and facial weakness. She has a history of cholesteatoma associated with foul smelling discharge. Which of the following is the most likely diagnosis?

(a)   Meningitis
(b)   Extradural abscess
(c)   Facial nerve palsy
(d)   Perforation of tympanic membrane
(e)   Lateral sinus thrombosis

8.   A 50-year-old man presents with halitosis and a 5 cm indistinct mass behind sternocleidomastoid muscle below the thyroid cartilage. The lump is soft, smooth and compressible on palpation. He is just recovering from a chest infection. Which of the following is the most likely diagnosis?

(a)   Pharyngeal pouch
(b)   Thyroglossal cyst
(c)   Cystic hygroma
(d)   Goitre
(e)   Metastatic carcinoma

9.   A 2-year-old girl presents with deafness and retinitis pigmentosa. Which of the following is the most likely syndrome?

(a)   Pendred's syndrome
(b)   Pierre-Robin sequence
(c)   Refsum syndrome
(d)   Treacher-Collins syndrome
(e)   Usher's syndrome

10. A 4-year-old boy from Bangladesh presents with a 2-month history of rapidly increasing left anterior triangle mass. Ultrasound reveals multiple, enlarged, conglomerating roundish lymph nodes that are hypoechoic. Chest X-ray, Heaf test, and full blood count are equivocal. The paediatricians have asked for a biopsy to rule out tuberculosis. What is the most appropriate treatment?

   (a) Excision lymph node biopsy
   (b) Incision lymph node biopsy
   (c) MDT discussion
   (d) Tonsillectomy
   (e) No surgery indicated

11. An 8-year-old girl presents with bilateral nasal polyps and frequent chest infections. Which of the following syndromes is most likely?

   (a) Burning mouth
   (b) CHARGE syndrome
   (c) Cystic fibrosis
   (d) Kartagener's syndrome
   (e) Young's syndrome

12. A 55-year-old musician presented with an intermittent neck swelling associated with hoarseness, cough and discomfort. Examination of the neck did not reveal any palpable mass but indirect laryngoscopy revealed fullness in the upper left hemilarynx. What is the most likely diagnosis?

   (a) Chronic laryngitis
   (b) Laryngocoele
   (c) Squamous cell carcinoma of larynx
   (d) Laryngeal papillomatosis
   (e) Keratosis of the vocal folds

13. What anatomical structure is innervated by the mandibular division of the trigeminal nerve?

   (a) Scutum
   (b) Sinus Tympani
   (c) Stapedius
   (d) Processus cochlearformis
   (e) Tensor Tympani

14. Salivary secretion is reduced in which of the following conditions?

   (a) Post-menopausal women
   (b) Pregnancy
   (c) Depression
   (d) Mouth ulcers
   (e) Pancreatitis

15. From which sub-division of the hypopharynx does the majority of tumours arise from?

   (a) Posterior pharyngel wall
   (b) Post cricoid
   (c) Piriform fossa
   (d) Cricoid cartilage
   (e) Vocal cord

16. Which of the following arteries is the main blood supply to glomus jugulare?

    (a) Facial artery
    (b) Ascending pharyngeal artery
    (c) Internal Maxillary artery
    (d) Lingual artery
    (e) Thyroid artery

17. An 18-year-old girl presents with a well-demarcated painful lesion on her uvula. What is the most likely diagnosis?

    (a) Squamous papilloma
    (b) Bullous pemphigoid
    (c) Syphilitic ulcer
    (d) Torus palatinus
    (e) Apthous ulcer

18. A 45-year-old diabetic woman presents with bilateral painless parotid swellings. What is the single most likely diagnosis?

    (a) Cheilitis glandularis
    (b) Sjogrens
    (c) Sialosis
    (d) Necrotizing sialometaplasia
    (e) Xerostomia

19. In which Le Fort fracture is CSF rhinorrhoea most common?

   (a)   I
   (b)   II
   (c)   III
   (d)   IV
   (e)   V

20. A 56-year-old man presents with 8mm mass on helix of right ear. The lesion is exquisitely painful and tender to touch. He now finds it uncomfortable to sleep on the right. On examination, the lesion is a well-defined raised lesion with crusting on top. When the crust is removed it reveals a channel. At the periphery, intact epidermis is edematous and acanthotic. Which of the following is the most likely diagnosis?

   (a)   Auricular endochondral pseudocyst
   (b)   Basal cell carcinoma
   (c)   Chondrodermatitis nodularis helicis
   (d)   Gouty tophi
   (e)   Keratoacanthoma

21. A 3-month-old boy presents with possible congenital hearing loss. Which of the following is the most appropriate diagnostic test?

   (a)   Auditory response cradle
   (b)   Pure tone audiogram
   (c)   Distraction testing
   (d)   Free field testing
   (e)   Tympanometry

22. What type of hypersensitivity reaction is involve in the Mantoux test?

    (a) I
    (b) II
    (c) III
    (d) IV
    (e) V

23. A 45-year-old male patient presents with a foreign body sensation in throat and intermittent voice break. Nasoendoscopy shows a unilateral midline mass arising from left vocal cord. Which of the following is the most likely diagnosis?

    (a) Reinke's oedema
    (b) Singers nodules
    (c) Vocal cord polyp
    (d) Acute laryngitis
    (e) Vocal Cord granuloma

24. Comparing DO-HNS exam scores between the north and south of England. What is the single most suitable statistical test?

    (a) Two sample (unpaired) Students t-test
    (b) Two way analysis of variance (ANOVA)
    (c) Wilcoxon matched pair test
    (d) One way analysis of variance
    (e) Mann-Whitney U Test

25. With regards the UK Guidelines in ENT practice for tonsillectomy and the selection criteria to consider surgery; what is the number of episodes of peritonsillar abscesses (quincies) required for listing a patient for bilateral tonsillectomies?

    (a)   1 episode
    (b)   2 episodes
    (c)   3 episodes
    (d)   4 episodes
    (e)   5 episodes

26. A 50-year-old woman presents with a painless, firm, neck swelling located on the right. Fine needle aspiration shows multiple compact follicles. After lobectomy histology shows evidence of capsular and blood vessel invasion. What is the most likely pathology?

    (a)   Follicular adenoma
    (b)   Follicular carcinoma
    (c)   Lymphoma
    (d)   Anaplastic carcinoma
    (e)   Medullary carcinoma

27. A 38-year-old man presents with normal symmetry and tone at rest but moderate-good forehead movement and complete eye closure with effort. Close inspection reveals only slight facial weakness. What is the House-Brackman (HB) grading of facial nerve palsy?

    (a)   HB Grade I
    (b)   HB Grade II
    (c)   HB Grade III
    (d)   HB Grade IV
    (e)   HB Grade V

28. What is the amount of adrenaline contained in 1ml of 1: 200,000 adrenaline solution?

(a) 5mcg
(b) 50mcg
(c) 500mcg
(d) 10mcg
(e) 100mcg

29. A 35-year-old man presents with unilateral conductive hearing loss. On examination has peduculated mass extending from the bony cartilaginous junction of the external auditory canal. What is the most likely diagnosis?

(a) Ear canal polyp
(b) Exostoses
(c) Osteoma
(d) Pyogenic granuloma
(e) Foreign body

30. A 25-year-old man presents with hearing loss after a falling from a ladder. Tympanometry reveals peak compliance is between -100 and +100 daPa but the reading was off the y-axis. What is the single most likely tympanogram?

(a) Type As
(b) Type Ad
(c) Type B
(d) Type C1
(e) Type C2

31. A 55 year old patient presents with a painless 5 x 6mm ulcerative lesion on superior border of the right pinna in the region of Darwin tubercle. Which is the most likely diagnosis?

    (a) Squamous cell carcinoma
    (b) Basal Cell Carcinoma
    (c) Melanoma
    (d) Chondrodermatitis nodularis helicis
    (e) Keratoacanthoma

32. A 56-year-old man presents with difficulty walking without holding onto something. He also claims that objects bounce up and down when he is in a car. He was recently admitted to hospital and received intravenous treatment for a bladder infection. Which of the following drugs is most likely to be responsible?

    (a) Frusemide
    (b) Neomycin
    (c) Gentamycin
    (d) Cisplatin
    (e) Aspirin

33. What is the best investigation to confirm a laryngeal cleft in a baby?

    (a) Microlaryngoscopy and Bronchoscopy
    (b) Barium swallow
    (c) Flexible nasendoscopy
    (d) X-ray
    (e) Radio-labelled milk swallow

34. A 45-year-old Chinese woman presents with epistaxis. Examination and biopsy reveals a nasopharyngeal carcinoma that extends into the nasal cavity and oropharynx. There is a unilateral neck node measuring 6cm in greatest dimension above the supraclavicular fossa. What is the TNM staging?

    a) T1N1M0
    b) T2N1M1
    c) T2N1M0
    d) T3N1M0
    e) T3N0M0

35. A 45-year-old woman presents with nystagmus which increases in intensity when she looks to the left and decreases on gaze to the right. She has a vestibular lesion on the left. What is the most relevant explanation?

    (a) Boyce's sign
    (b) Tullio phenomena
    (c) Alexander's law
    (d) Arnold's reflex
    (e) Grisel sign

36. A 35-year-old man presents with an acute facial pain. He also describes a preceding aura of flashing lights and has had a number of similar episodes in the past. What is the most likely diagnosis?

    (a) Herpes zoster
    (b) Ramsay Hunt syndrome
    (c) Migraine
    (d) Sinusitis
    (e) Trigeminal neuralgia

37. A 75 year old man presents with left sided headache associated with tenderness over the scalp, jaw claudication, fever and visual changes. Which statement is most accurate?

    (a) The condition responds well to caffeine-free diet and ergotamine
    (b) The appropriate treatment is 1 week course of high dose of steroids
    (c) ESR and CRP are elevated
    (d) Temporal artery biopsy is diagnostic in 90% of cases
    (e) The condition is more common in males than females

38. What volume of saline is needed to make a solution containing 200mg of 5% cocaine?

    (a) 2mls
    (b) 4mls
    (c) 10mls
    (d) 20mls
    (e) 40mls

39. A 10-year-old boy presents with a preauricular sinus and mucoid discharge from a small pit in his neck. He is under the care of the renal physician. Investigations reveal bilaterally sensorineural deafness. What is the most likely syndrome in this case?

    (a) Alport
    (b) Alstrom
    (c) Branchia-Oto-Renal
    (d) CHARGE
    (e) Waardenburg

40.   From which branchial pouch are the superior parathyroids
        embryologically derived?

        (a)   First pouch
        (b)   Second pouch
        (c)   Third pouch
        (d)   Fourth pouch
        (e)   Sixth pouch

41.   A 27-year-old woman presents with a butterfly-shaped rash
        over her face and joint pain in her hands. Flexible
        nasendoscopic examination revealed nasopharyngeal
        ulceration. What is the most likely diagnosis?

        (a)   Relapsing polychondritis
        (b)   Sjögren's syndrome
        (c)   Syphilis
        (d)   Systemic lupus erythematous
        (e)   Tuberculosis

42.   Which of the following airway noises is a sign of
        laryngomalacia?

        (a)   Stertor
        (b)   Low pitched inspiratory stridor
        (c)   Low pitched expiratory stridor
        (d)   High pitched inspiratory stridor
        (e)   High pitched expiratory stridor

43. A 60-year-old woman presents with unilateral deafness and tinnitus for many years. On examination there is an absent corneal reflex and ataxia. What is the most likely diagnosis?

    (a) Acoustic neuroma
    (b) Cholesteatoma
    (c) Otoclerosis
    (d) Otosyphilis
    (e) Otospongiosis

44. Acute mastoiditis affects which age group predominantly?

    (a) <1 year
    (b) <2 years
    (c) 5-10 years
    (d) 10-40 years
    (e) >50 years

45. A 45-year-old female presents with a low frequency sensorineural hearing loss noted on pure tone audiogram. She has normal tympanometry and stapedial reflexes. What is the most likely diagnosis?

    (a) Menieres disease
    (b) Waadenburg syndrome type I
    (c) Waardenburg syndrome type IV
    (d) Pendred syndrome
    (e) Presbyacusis

46. A 40-year-old woman presents with a feeling of "lightheadedness' whenever she goes to a shopping mall. She has to sit down to recover and often complains of tingling in her fingers. When eating out at resturants, she feels comfortable near the door rather than in the centre of the room. What is the most likely diagnosis?

    (a) Migraine
    (b) BPPV
    (c) Psychogenic
    (d) Acute labyrinthitis
    (e) Vertebro-basilar ischaemia

47. Visual analogue scale responses of a group of subjects (n = 16) who were asked to report their perceived contentment on 2 consectutive days. Which is the most suitable statistical test?

    (a) Wilcoxon matched pairs test
    (b) Mann-Whitney U test
    (c) Chi-Squared (X2) test
    (d) One Sample (paired) Student's t-test
    (e) Two sample (unpaired) Student's t- test

48. Epistaxis is associated with which of the following condition(s)?

    (a) Hereditary familial telangiectasia (Osler-Weber-Rendu)
    (b) Foreign body
    (c) Leukaemia
    (d) Anti-platelet drugs
    (e) All of the above

49. A 50-year-old female patient present with a two-year history of hoarse voice and some difficulty breathing. Examination reveals a bluish colouration on her nose and flexible nasendoscopy shows a smooth benign looking supraglottic lesion. Blood tests reveal calcium of 3.8mmol/L. What is the most likely diagnosis?

   (a) Wegener's
   (b) Sarcoidosis
   (c) Hyperthyroidism
   (d) Churg-Strauss syndrome
   (e) Tuberculosis

50. An 8-year-old son of a Jehovah's Witness is brought to hospital with a post tonsillectomy bleed. It fails to settle with conservative measures. He requires a transfusion and return to theatre. Both parents refuse to consent for either. Which of the following statements is the most appropriate next step?

   (a) Make patient ward of court
   (b) Obtain consent from an alternative next of kin
   (c) Obtain consent from the patient
   (d) Surgery & transfusion proceed without consent
   (e) Surgery can proceed after promising to the parents that you will not give a blood transfusion

51. Which instrument is used to give full exposure to the oropharynx for tonsillectomy?

   (a) Mollison's pillar retractor
   (b) Negus laryngoscope
   (c) Jolls retractor
   (d) Travers retractor
   (e) Boyle's-Davis

52. A 35-year-old man who has had subcutaneous Vicryl sutures used to close his wound after a total thyroidectomy. What would you advise him?

(a) Do not immerse in water
(b) Gargle saline
(c) Avoid contact sports
(d) Stop smoking
(e) Continue as before

53. Frontal sinus is supplied by which artery?

(a) Sphenopalatine artery
(b) Greater palatine artery
(c) Labial artery
(d) Anterior ethmoidal artery
(e) Posterior ethmoidal artery

54. Congenital nasal midline lesions are rare. What would be the most appropriate initial management?

(a) Conservative period of observation
(b) Examination and biopsy
(c) CT scan
(d) MRI scan
(e) CT and MRI scans

55. A 5-year-old boy presents with a swelling near the glabella that has been present since birth. It has a pit and is firm to palpation. What is the most likely diagnosis?

   (a) Basal cell carcinoma
   (b) Haemangioma
   (c) Nasoaveolar cyst
   (d) Nasal dermoid
   (e) Nasal glioma

56. A 37 year old man presents with a unilateral nasal mass, which on biopsy is diagnosed as esthesioneuroblastoma. The lesion appears to penetrate the skull base to the dura but it does not penetrate the dura. The best therapy for this patient is

   (a) Chemoradiation therapy
   (b) Radiation therapy followed by surgery
   (c) Surgery followed by radiation therapy
   (d) Endoscopic debulking and radiation therapy
   (e) Chemoradiation therapy and palliative therapy

57. Which of the following statement pertaining to TORCH perinatal infections is incorrect?

(a) Rubella and Varicella –Zoster infection may be treated with antiviral agents
(b) The 'other agents' included under O include Hep B virus, Varicella –Zoster virus, Coxsackie virus, syphilis and HIV.
(c) Hearing impairment mental retardation, autism and death may be caused by TORCH infection
(d) Some TORCH infections can be effective treated with antibiotics if the mother is diagnosed early in pregnancy or prevented by vaccination.
(e) Sabre-tibia is a recognized condition associated with TORCH infection

58. A 8-year-old-girl is referred with periorbital cellulitis. You examined her and found no visual defect in acuity or colour vision. Eye movements and light reflexes were normal and there is no proptosis or ptosis. You diagnose preseptal cellulitis. What is your initial management?

(a) CT scan
(b) Nasal congestant
(c) IV augmentin
(d) IV benzylpenicillin
(e) IV Amoxicillin

59. A 45-year-old man presents with a right sided facial nerve palsy (House-Brackman grade 4). He states that prior to the facial weakness he had a dull ache in the right ear. He also had a history of itching and discharge from both ears. Examination revealed normal tympanic membranes and canals with flaky skin on both sides. What is the most likely diagnosis?

    (a) Active squamous chronic otitis media
    (b) Bells palsy
    (c) Herpes zoster
    (d) Lyme disease
    (e) Sarcoidosis

60. Human papilloma virus (HPV) is a DNA virus. Types 6 and 11 are responsible mainly for recurrent respiratory papillomatosis. Which of the following can be considered for the prevention of types 6 and 11?

    (a) Aciclovir
    (b) Valaciclovir
    (c) Podofilox or Condylox
    (d) Cervarix vaccine
    (e) Gardasil vaccine

61. A 4-year-old girl presents with a discharge above the left tragus. Examination reveals a preauricular sinus. Which branchial arch is most likely to be responsible?

    (a) First branchial arch
    (b) Second branchial arch
    (c) Third branchial arch
    (d) Fourth branchial arch
    (e) Sixth branchial arch

62. What are the chemical components of BIPP?

   (a) Iodoform, benzoin & storax
   (b) Iodoform, Paraffin & Bismuth
   (c) Fluticasone fuorate & iodine
   (d) Fluticasone proprionate & iodine
   (e) Ipratropium bromide & iodine

63. The maxillary nerve passes through which of the following anatomical openings to exit the cranial vault.

   (a) Superior orbital fissure
   (b) Foramen Ovale
   (c) Foramen Rotundum
   (d) Foramen Spinosum
   (e) Foramen Lacerum

64. What is the bony landmark for the anterior branch of the middle meningeal artery?

   (a) Asterion
   (b) Bregma
   (c) Inion
   (d) Rhinion
   (e) Pterion

65. Which structure within the cochlear separates the scala media from the scala tympani?

   (a) Reissner's membrane
   (b) Basilar membrane
   (c) Organ of Corti
   (d) Oval window
   (e) Helicotrema

66. Which immunoglobulin is responsible for secondary immune response?

  (a) IgA
  (b) IgD
  (c) IgG
  (d) IgE
  (e) IgM

67. With regards study validation, which one of the following statements is true?

  (a) Specificity indicates how good the test is at picking up people who have the condition
  (b) Sensitivity indicates how good the test is at correctly excluding people without the condition
  (c) The negative predictive value (NPV) is the pre test probability that if a person's test is negative, that he or she has the disease
  (d) Positive predictive value (PPV) is the post test probability of a positive result and is the probability of someone having the disease if they have a positive test result
  (e) The prevalence of the condition is the number with disease in the sample size of the population size

68. Which metabolic abnormality is most likely in a patient who underwent pharyngo-laryngectomy with stomach interposition complicated by acute tubular necrosis?

  (a) hypokalaemia
  (b) hyperkalaemia
  (c) hypercalcaemia
  (d) hypernatraemia
  (e) hyponatraemia

69. Which test is the most specific for Granulomatosis with polyangiitis (GPA), formerly known as Wegener's granulomatosis?

(a) p-ANCA
(b) c-ANCA
(c) PR9
(d) ACE
(e) ANA

70. A 39-year-old woman presents complaining of paraesthesia on the medial aspect of the forearm 2 weeks after neck dissection. Which nerve has most likely been damaged?

(a) C6
(b) C7
(c) C8
(d) T1
(e) T2

71. A 10-year-old Greek boy presents for genetic screening because of anaemia. The result reveals a common single gene disorder. What is the most likely genetic condition?

(a) Klinefelter syndrome
(b) Thalassaemia trait
(c) Haemophila A
(d) Prader-Willi syndrome
(e) Osteogenesis imperfecta

72. Which investigation provides definitive diagnosis for achalasia?

(a) X-Ray
(b) Ultrasound scan
(c) CT scan
(d) Endoscopy
(e) Oesophageal manometry

73. A Pharyngeal pouch emerges between which muscles?

(a) Cricothyroid and inferior constrictor
(b) cricopharyngeus and thyropharyngeus
(c) Superior and inferior constrictor
(d) Thyrohyoid and middle constrictor
(e) Middle constrictor and thyropharyngeus

74. A 47-year-old man presents with a 5 x 4 cm neck mass below the level of the hyoid bone. The lump first appeared following a kick in the neck during a rugby match. He was reassured by a casualty senior house officer that it would go away with time as it was most likely to be a haematoma. It persisted and became infected twice requiring antibiotics. On examination it does not move on swallowing or on tongue protrusion. Ultrasound scanning reveals a cystic lesion. Which of the following is the most likely cause for the neck mass?

(a) Anaplastic thyroid cancer
(b) Medullary thyroid carcinoma
(c) Papillary thyroid carcinoma
(d) Thyroglossal cyst
(e) Dermoid cyst

75. Which of the following nerve is at risk during dissection in the sterno-thyro-laryngeal (Joll's) triangle:

    (a) Recurrent laryngeal nerve
    (b) External branch of the superior laryngeal nerve
    (c) Internal branch of the superior laryngeal nerve
    (d) Vagus
    (e) Hypoglossal nerve

76. Which cranial nerve innervates the anterior belly of digastrics?

    (a) Facial nerve
    (b) Trigeminal nerve
    (c) Hypoglossal nerve
    (d) Vagus nerve
    (e) Glossopharyngeal nerve

77. The maximum safe dose of which local anaesthetic agent is 2mg/kg (without adrenaline).

    (a) Bupivacaine
    (b) Cocaine
    (c) Levobupivacaine
    (d) Lignocaine
    (e) Prilocaine

78. A 27-year-old woman presents with deafness following her pregnancy. Otoscopy reveals a pink tinge behind the tympanic membrane. Which is the most likely eponymous name?

(a) Hitselberger's sign
(b) Schwartze's sign
(c) Aquino's sign
(d) Brown's sign
(e) Hennebert's sign

79. A 16-year-old male presents with a 6 month history of severe day time somnolence. He has frequent day time naps but they do not make him feel more refreshed. He sleeps 12 hours at night and wakes up, when forced, still feeling tired. Polysomnography is normal. What is the most likely diagnosis?

(a) Periodic limb movement disorder
(b) Narcolepsy
(c) Upper airways resistance syndrome
(d) Central sleep apnoea
(e) Idiopathic hypersomnolence

80. Which of the following is incorrect regarding Naseptin?

(a) It contains mupirocin
(b) It is a cream rather than an ointment
(c) It may cause hypersensitivity reaction with long term usage
(d) It contains arachnis oil
(e) It has antibacterial properties

81. Which of the following statement is true regarding Xylometazoline?

   (a) It is a alpha adrenergic antagonist
   (b) It is a beta adrenergic antagonist
   (c) It is less effective after prolonged use
   (d) It is a beta adrenergic agonist
   (e) It can be used in children under 5 years

82. With regards lymphatic drainage of the head and neck region; the palatine tonsils and lateral oropharyngeal wall drain into which of these nodes?

   (a) Jugulo-omohyoid nodes
   (b) Jugulo-digastric nodes
   (c) Submandibular nodes
   (d) Anterior cervical nodes
   (e) Internal jugular nodes

83. A 38-year-old woman presents with a thyroid swelling. Fine needle aspiration cytology suggests a follicular thyroid lesion. Which is the most appropriate Thy staging?

   (a) Thy1
   (b) Thy2
   (c) Thy3
   (d Thy4
   (e) Thy5

84. A 49-year-old male obese patient presents complaining of snoring. His wife reports that he stops breathing several times each night for over 10 seconds. His sleep study reveals severe obstructive sleep apnoea with an AHI of 38. What would be the most appropriate management option?

    (a) Continuous positive airway pressure (CPAP)
    (b) Laser Assisted Uvuloplasty
    (c) Diathermy Assisted Uvuloplasty
    (d) Adenotonsillectomy
    (e) Tracheostomy

85. A 65-year-old male patient presents with dysphagia and a mass in the neck that gurgle on palpation. What is the most likely diagnosis?

    (a) Boyce's sign
    (b) Bryce sign
    (c) Alexander's law
    (d) Arnold's reflex
    (e) Grisel sign

86. A 4-year-old boy presents with first presentation of bilateral conductive hearing loss secondary to glue ear. What is the most appropriate management?

    (a) Repeat hearing test with 6 week time interval
    (b) Repeat hearing test in 3 months
    (c) Recommend hearing aids
    (d) Insert grommets
    (e) Insert grommets and adenoidectomy

87.   A 59-year-old Asian man presents with a history of nasal
        obstruction and epistaxis. CT scanning shows a mass in the
        left ethmoid sinus invading the orbit but not the extending
        intracranially. There are no neck nodes. What is the TNM
        stage?

        (a)   T2N0M0
        (b)   T2N1M0
        (c)   T3N0M0
        (d)   T3N1M0
        (e)   T4N1M0

88.   A 14-year-old boy presents with progressive sensorineural
        hearing loss, which suddenly worsens following head
        trauma whilst playing rugby. Which of the following is the
        most appropriate diagnosis?

        (a)   Benign intracranial hypertension
        (b)   Cochlear hydrops
        (c)   Enlarged vestibular aqueduct syndrome
        (d)   Mondini inner ear deformity
        (e)   Usher's syndrome

89.   A 78-year-old female patient sits up in bed with eyes wide
        open, answers questions but is not making sense. What is
        her GCS (Glasgow Coma Score)?

        (a)   11
        (b)   12
        (c)   13
        (d)   14
        (e)   15

90. What is the gold standard investigation for pharyngeal pouch?

    (a) Flexible nasendoscopy
    (b) Lateral soft tissue neck XR
    (c) USS neck
    (d) Barium swallow
    (e) CT with contrast

91. Cholesteatoma formation involves mainly the pars flaccida and negative middle ear pressure. Which theory best describes which theory of the aetiopathogenesis of acquired cholesteatoma?

    (a) Retraction pocket
    (b) Epidermoid formation
    (c) Epithelial migration
    (d) Iatrogenic or post-traumatic
    (e) Inflammation

92. A 52-year-old female presents with unilateral pulsatile tinnitus and conductive hearing loss. CT scan with contrast shows a vascular mass filling the epitypanum and mastoid cavity. What is the most likely diagnosis?

    (a) Patulous Eustachian tube
    (b) Palatal myoclonus
    (c) Glomus tympanicum
    (d) Venous malformation
    (e) Superior semicircular canal dehiscence

93. A 17-year-old female presents with hay fever and asthma complains of nasal and conjunctival   pruritis, sneezing and rhinorrhoea. What is the most likely diagnosis?

   (a)   Atrophic rhinitis
   (b)   Allergic rhinitis
   (c)   Drug induced rhinitis
   (d)   Hormonal rhinitis
   (e)   Non allergic occupational rhinitis

94. A 19 year old woman presents with itchy ears. A microbiological swab is taken and the report came   back stating a bacterium that commonly colonises human skin and mucosa. What is the most likely pathogen?

   (a)   Streptococcus pneumonia
   (b)   Streptococcus milleri
   (c)   Haemophilus influenza
   (d)   Staphylococcus aureus
   (e)   Pseudomonas aeruginosa

95. Which one of the following statements about atypical mycobacteria is true?

   (a)   The commonest species is Mycobacteria scrofulaceum
   (b)   Mycolymphadenitis affects mainly teenagers
   (c)   Lymphadenitis is painful
   (d)   Is treated with anti-TB medications for 4 weeks
   (e)   Surgical excision is curative in over 90% of cases

96. A child visits his grandfather who live on a rural farm with cattles. The child develops a skin rash, mouth ulcers and diarrhoea following the visit. Culture shows Brucellosis. The most likely mode of transmission of the disease is:

(a) From coming in contact with animals
(b) From drinking unpasteurised milk
(c) From coming in contact with other villagers
(d) From the soil
(e) From mosquitoes

97. Which nerve is mainly responsible for taste?

(a) Trigeminal nerve
(b) Lingual nerve
(c) Facial nerve
(d) Hypoglossal nerve
(e) Glossopharyngeal nerve

98. What is the most common tumour of the salivary glands?

(a) Hyalinizing clear cell carcinoma
(b) Epithelial-myoepithelial carcinoma
(c) Pleomorphic adenoma
(d) Acinic cell carcinoma
(e) Adenoid cystic carcinoma

99. A 49-year-old man presents complaining of asymmetrical tonsils. On examination he was found to have a medially displaced right tonsil. A CT scan report stated that he had a solid lesion in the post-styloid compartment of his parapharyngeal space. What is the most likely diagnosis?

   (a) Metastatic lesion
   (b) Salivary gland lesion
   (c) Neurogenic lesion
   (d) Lymphoma
   (e) Primary tonsillar lesion

100. Which is the correct botox treatment of Frey's syndrome?

   (a) 10u/cm of botox subcutaneously
   (b) 1u/cm botox intradermally
   (c) 1u/cm botox intraparotid
   (d) 1u/cm botox subcutaneously
   (e) 10u/cm botox intramuscularly

101. Which receptors are associated with rhinitis medicamentosa?

   (a) Alpha and H1
   (a) Beta and H1
   (b) Delta and H1
   (c) Alpha and Beta
   (d) Alpha, Beta and Delta

102. A 35-year-old male company director complains of difficulty hearing in the presence of background noises. His pure tone audiometry reveals moderate hearing loss at 250 Hz but the thresholds at the other frequencies are all less than 20 dBHL. What is the most appropriate initial hearing device?

    (a) In-the-canal (ITC) hearing aid
    (b) In-the-ear (ITE) hearing aid
    (c) Body-worn hearing aid
    (d) Bone anchored hearing aid
    (e) No device

103. A 25-year-old man presents with gradual blockage of both nostrils. The GP examined the nose and noted pale insensate swellings bilaterally. The patient is also asthmatic and sensitive to aspirin. What is the most likely diagnosis?

    (a) Nasolabial cyst
    (b) Nasal polyps
    (c) Nasopharyngeal carcinoma
    (d) Mucocoele
    (e) Encephalocoele

104. A 65-year-old woman presents with asymmetrical sensory neural hearing loss without tinnitus. Which of the following is the most appropriate imaging modality?

    (a) CT scan with contrast
    (b) Gadolinium enhanced MRI scan
    (c) MRI STIR sequence
    (d) MRI non echo planar diffusion weighted
    (e) FDG PET CT

105. A 26-year-old male presents with recurrent acute left maxillary sinusitis. CT scan shows opacification within left antrum. What is the most appropriate treatment?

   (a) Balloon sinuplasty
   (b) Antral washout
   (c) Turbinate surgery
   (d) SMD Inferior Turbinates
   (e) Functional Endoscopic Sinus Surgery

106. What is the most appropriate genetic description for one of the alternative versions of a gene that can occupy a specific locus?

   (a) Genotype
   (b) Phenotype
   (c) Mosaicism
   (d) Allele
   (e) Meiosis

107. A 56-year-old man presents with a bilateral symmetrical sensorineural loss showing a virtually flat line across all frequencies and well-preserved speech discrimination. What is the single most likely diagnosis?

   (a) Cogan's syndrome
   (b) Inner ear condudive presbyacusis
   (c) Neural presbyacusis
   (d) Sensory presbyacusis
   (e) Strial presbyacusis

108. A 76-year-old man present underwent unilateral resection of the upper jaw for carcinoma of the maxillary sinus. He requires a biomaterial to support the soft tissues of the cheek. What is the most appropriate biomaterial?

   (a)   Gutta percha
   (b)   Hydrozyapatite
   (c)   Medpore
   (d)   Ceramic
   (e)   Teflon

109. A 5-year-old boy presents to his GP with inflamed tonsils and pyrexia of 37.5 C after 7 days with a sore throat. He is able to eat and drink. Blood test reveals a neutrophilia. Which antibiotic therapy would be the most appropriate?

   (a)   Oral Penicillin V
   (b)   Oral Metronidazole
   (c)   Oral Co-Amoxiclav
   (d)   IV Benzylpenicillin
   (e)   IV Co-Amoxiclav

110. Which definition best describes the hiatus semilunaris?

   (a)   A two dimensional space between the uncinate process and the bulla ethmoidalis
   (b)   A three dimesional space between the uncinate process, the bulla ethmoidalis and the lamina papyracea
   (c)   A three dimensional space between the agger nasi cell, ground lamella and the lamina papyracea
   (d)   A two dimensional space between the uncinate process and the middle turbinate
   (e)   A two dimensional space between the uncinate and the haller cell

111. A 4-year-old boy presents with sudden onset noisy breathing and drooling. The child appears scared, flushed and stridulous. On examination, he is noted to be in a tripod position, pyrexial and using accessory muscles during respiration. What is the likely diagnosis?

(a) Allergic reaction
(b) Acute tonsillitis
(c) Acute epiglottitis
(d) Acute laryngotracheobronchitis (croup)
(e) Vocal cord palsy

112. The fundamental difference between paroxysmal hemicrania and cluster headache is...

(a) Ptosis
(b) Rhinorrhoea
(c) Nasal obstruction
(d) Unilateral pain
(e) Response to indometacin

PAPER TWO		
Answers		
1.	E	Down syndrome
2.	C	Case control study
3.	A	T1N0M0
4.	E	Syphilis
5.	C	Horizontal to the left
6.	A	Michel aplasia
7.	B	Extradural abscess
8.	A	Pharyngeal pouch
9.	E	Usher's syndrome
10.	A	Excision lymph node biopsy
11.	C	Cystic fibrosis
12.	B	Laryngocoele
13.	E	Tensor tympani
14.	C	Depression
15.	C	Piriform fossa
16.	B	Ascending pharyngeal artery
17.	A	Squamous papilloma
18.	C	Sialosis
19.	C	III
20.	C	Chondrodermatitis nodularis helicis
21.	A	Auditory response cradle
22.	D	IV
23.	C	Vocal cord polyp
24.	E	Mann-Whitney U Test
25.	B	2 episodes
26.	B	Follicular carcinoma
27.	B	HB Grade II
28.	A	5mcg
29.	C	Osteoma

30.	B	Type Ad
31.	B	Basal cell carcinoma
32.	C	Gentamicin
33.	A	Microlaryngoscopy and Bronchoscopy
34.	C	T2N1M0
35.	C	Alexander's law
36.	C	Migraine
37.	D	Temporal artery biopsy is diagnostic in 90% of cases
38.	B	4mls
39.	C	Branchi-oto-renal
40.	D	Fourth pouch
41.	D	Systemic lupus erythematous
42.	B	Low pitched inspiratory stridor
43.	A	Acoustic neuroma
44.	B	<2 yrs
45.	A	Meniere's disease
46.	C	Psychogenic
47.	A	Wilcoxon matched pairs test
48.	E	All of the above
49.	B	Sarcoidosis
50.	A	Make patient ward of court
51.	E	Boyle-Davis
52.	A	Do not immerse in water *(vicyl is broken down by hydrolysis – the splitting of covalent bonds by water)*
53.	D	Anterior ethmoidal artery
54.	E	CT & MRI scans
55.	D	Nasal dermoid
56.	C	Surgery followed by radiation therapy
57.	A	Rubella and Varicella –Zoster infection may be treated with antiviral agents
58.	C	IV Augmentin

59.	B	Bells palsy
60.	E	Gardasil vaccine
61.	A	First branchial arch
62.	B	Iodoform paraffin bismuth
63.	C	Foramen rotundum
64.	E	Pterion
65.	B	Basilar membrane
66.	C	IgG
67.	D	Positive predictive value (PPV) is the post test probability of a positive result and is the probability of someone having the disease if they have a positive test result
68.	B	Hyperkalaemia
69.	B	c-ANCA
70.	D	T1
71.	B	Thalassaemia trait
72.	E	Oesophageal manometry
73.	B	cricopharyngeus and thyropharyngeus
74.	D	Thyroglossal cyst
75.	B	External branch of the superior laryngeal nerve
76.	B	Trigeminal nerve
77.	A	Bupivicaine
78.	B	Schwartze's sign
79.	E	Idiopathic hypersomnolence
80.	A	It contains mupirocin
81.	C	It is less effective after prolonged use
82.	B	Jugulo-digastric nodes
83.	C	Thy 3
84.	A	Continuous positive airway pressure (CPAP)
85.	A	Boyce's sign
86.	B	Repeat hearing test in 3 months

87.	C	T3N0M0
88.	C	Enlarged vestibular aqueduct syndrome
89.	D	14
90.	D	Barium swallow
91.	A	Retraction pocket theory
92.	C	Glomus tympanicum
93.	B	Allergic rhinitis
94.	D	Staphylococcus aureus
95.	E	Surgical excision is curative in over 90% of cases
96.	B	From drinking unpasteurised milk
97.	C	Facial nerve *(chorda tympani)*
98.	C	Pleomorphic adenoma
99.	C	Neurogenic lesion
100.	B	1u/cm botox intradermally
101.	C	Alpha & Beta
102.	E	No device
103.	B	Nasal polyps *(Samter's tria: polyps, asthma and aspirin hypersensitivity)*
104.	B	Gadolinium enhanced MRI scan
105.	E	Functional endoscopic sinus surgery
106.	D	Allele
107.	E	Strial presbyacusis
108.	A	Gutta percha
109.	A	Oral Penicillin V
110.	A	A two dimensional space between the uncinate process and the bulla ethmoidalis
111.	C	Acute epiglottitis
112.	E	Response to indometacin

1. Which syndrome is characterised by incomplete development of one ear?

    (a) Down syndrome
    (b) Goldenhar syndrome
    (c) Promin auris
    (d) Treacher-collins
    (e) Cri-du-chat syndrome

2. Which of the following is the best explanation of Frey's Syndrome following parotid surgery?

    (a) Parasympathetic parotid nerve fibres connecting with sympathetic sweat gland fibres using acetylcholine as the neurotransmitter.
    (b) Sympathetic parotid nerve fibres connecting with parasympathetic sweat gland fibres using adrenaline as the neurotransmitter.
    (c) Parasympathetic parotid nerve fibres connecting with sympathetic sweat gland fibres using noradrenaline as the neurotransmitter
    (d) Sympathetic parotid nerve fibres connecting with parasympathetic sweat gland fibres using noradrenaline as the neurotransmitter.
    (e) Parasympathetic parotid nerve fibres connecting with parasympathetic sweat gland fibres using acetylcholine as the neurotransmitter

3. Which segment of the facial nerve is damaged if lacrimation and stapedial reflex are preserved but facial movements and taste to the anterior 2/3 of the tongue are absent?

    (a) Meatal
    (b) Labyrinthine
    (c) Tympanic
    (d) Mastoid
    (e) Extracranial

4. What treatment option is inappropriate for the management of rhinitis medicimentosa?

    (a) Oxymethazoline spray
    (b) Nasonex spray
    (c) Flixonase spray
    (d) Saline nasal douching
    (e) Short course of oral steroids

5. In an observational cohort study of treatment of sinusitis, patients are treated with either antibiotics or surgery. Failure to recognize that the patients who receive surgical intervention generally have more severe symptoms represents a problem with:

    (a) Selection bias
    (b) Confounding bias
    (c) Detection bias
    (d) Comorbidity bias
    (e) Intervention bias

6.   Which of the following is a symptom of vestibular disorder?

(a)   Vomiting
(b)   Panic attacks
(c)   Imbalance
(d)   Faintness
(e)   Muzzy / fuzzy head

7.   A 50-year-old man present with a painless swelling in the upper lateral part of his neck on the left side deep to and protruding from the anterior upper 1/3 of sternocleidomastoid muscle. It measured 5 cm in diameter and was smooth, non-tender and fluctuant. Which of the following is the most likely diagnosis?

(a)   Cystic hygroma
(b)   Branchial cyst
(c)   Sternomastoid tumour
(d)   Thyroglossal cyst
(e)   Glomus jugular tumour

8.   Which skull base foramen permits entry of the middle meningeal artery to the cranium?

(a)   Foramen Ovale
(b)   Foramen Rotundum
(c)   Foramen Spinosum
(d)   Foramen Lacerum
(e)   Jugular foramen

9. A 46-year-old man presents with a 3 month history of a rapidly enlarging level 2 lymph node. Has had night sweats, fever and weight loss. The node is painful when he drinks alcohol. ENT examination is otherwise normal. Fine needle cytology of the lymph node shows atypical lymphocytes but cannot rule out lymphoma. What is the most appropriate treatment?

   (a) Excision lymph node biopsy
   (b) Incision lymph node biopsy
   (c) MDT discussion
   (d) Tonsillectomy
   (e) No surgery indicated

10. A 56-year-old male smoker presents with hoarse and weak voice that gets winded when trying to speak long sentences. Which of the following is the most likely diagnosis?

   (a) Acute laryngitis
   (b) Essential tremor
   (c) Reinke's oedema
   (d) Singer's nodules
   (e) Vocal cord palsy

11. Stapedius tendon exits from which anatomical structure to attach to stapes?

   (a) Petrotympanic fissure
   (b) Facial recess
   (c) Prussac's space
   (d) Pyramidal eminence
   (e) Stylomastoid formamen

12. Which structure / structures articulate with the cricoid cartilage?

   (a) Epiglottis
   (b) Thyroid cartilage
   (c) Arytenoids
   (d) Thyroid cartilage & arytenoids
   (e) Epiglottis & arytenoids

13. A 46-year-old woman presents with a blue, translucent swelling in the floor of her mouth. Which of the following is the most likely diagnosis?

   (a) Mikullicz's syndrome
   (b) syndrome
   (c) Oncocytoma
   (d) Mucous retention cyst
   (e) Ranula
   (f) Acute sialadenitis

14. Which bony landmark is important for mastoid surgery?

   (a) Inion
   (b) Pterion
   (c) Spine of Henle
   (d) Tympanic ring
   (e) Tympano-mastoid suture

15. In a study of pain following tonsillectomy, patients were randomly allocated to receive either an analgesia or placebo 2 hours pre-operatively. All patients were asked to rate their pain 2 hours after surgery using the scale: 0=no pain, 1=mild, 2=moderate, 3=severe. Which would be the most suitable statistical test?

    (a) Pearsons correlation coefficient
    (b) Spearmans rank correlation coefficient
    (c) Chi-Squared (X2) test
    (d) Mann-Whitney U Test
    (e) Wilcoxon matched pairs test

16. Which of the following statements about oral cavity pathology is CORRECT:

    (a) Lichen planus is usually a unilateral finding that responds well to laser ablation
    (b) A non-tender midline hard swelling of the hard palate is most often a minor salivary gland tumour
    (c) Erosive lichen planus is not associated with malignant transformation
    (d) Median rhomboid glossitis is best treated with antifungal lozenges
    (e) Leukoplakia and erythroplakia are equally pre-malignant conditions

17. An 18-year-old girl presents with a mass which appeared on the lobule of her left ear. It is mobile under the skin and recently became red and tender. Which of the following is the most likely diagnosis?

   (a) Auricular endochondral pseudocyst
   (b) Sebaceous cyst
   (c) Chondrodermatitis nodularis helicis
   (d) Gouty tophi
   (e) Pinna cellulitis

18. An 8-month-old girl presents with suspicion of hearing loss. Which of the following is the most appropriate diagnostic test?

   (a) Auditory response cradle
   (b) Pure tone audiogram
   (c) Distraction testing
   (d) Free field testing
   (e) Tympanometry

19. A 48-year-old woman presents with oral ulcers. Immunological investigations reveal antibodies to desmoglein 3. What is the most likely diagnosis?

   (a) Erythema multiforme
   (b) Pemphigoid
   (c) Pemphigus
   (d) Hereditary angio-oedema
   (e) Median Rhomboid glossitis

20. A 25-year-old man presents with hearing loss. Audiometry was consistent with otosclerosis. What is the single most likely tympanogram?

   (a) Type As
   (b) Type Ad
   (c) Type B
   (d) Type C1
   (e) Type C2

21. A 8-year-old boy presents with recurrent tonsillitis. His mother gives a history of heavy snoring but no witnessed apnoeic episodes. There is no daytime somnolence or irritability. He has had 4 attacks of tonsillitis a year for the last 2 years. What is the most appropriate treatment?

   (a) Tonsillectomy
   (b) Adenoidectomy
   (c) Adenotonsillectomy
   (d) SMD inferior turbinates
   (e) No surgery indicated

22. What is the most likely corresponding eponymous name for an air cell related to the maxillary sinus?

   (a) Haller cells
   (b) Kuhn cells
   (c) Kupffer cells
   (d) Onodi cells
   (e) Schwann cells

23. A 32-year-old woman presents with increasing weight gain, lethargy and neck swelling. On examination the patient has a firm rubbery goitre. Fine needle aspiration shows a diffuse lymphocytic/plasma cell infiltrate with the presence of lymphoid follicles and parenchymal atrophy. What is the most appropriate pathology?

   (a) Follicular adenoma
   (b) Follicular carcinoma
   (c) Lymphoma
   (d) Anaplastic carcinoma
   (e) Medullary carcinoma

24. A 38-year-old man presents with no facial movements present. What is the House-Brackman (HB) grading of facial nerve palsy?

   (a) HB Grade I
   (b) HB Grade II
   (c) HB Grade V
   (d) HB Grade VI
   (e) HB Grade VII

25. A 69-year-old female presents with severe bilateral otalgia and conductive hearing loss. Otoscopy shows widened EAC medially, thickened tympanic membrane and hyperaemic skin with granulation tissue. What is the most likely diagnosis?

   (a) Keratosis Obturans
   (b) Necrotizing otitis externa
   (c) Canal stenosis or atresia
   (d) Otitis externa
   (e) Squamous cell carcinoma of the external auditory canal

26. What is the maximum air bone gap possible?

    (a)   20 dB HL
    (b)   40 dB HL
    (c)   50 dB HL
    (d)   60 dB HL
    (e)   80 dB HL

27. An 80-year-old man presents with a pearly edged lesion on the vertex of his scalp. He is a regular golfer. What is the most likely diagnosis?

    (a)   Acral lentiginous melanoma
    (b)   Basal cell carcinoma
    (c)   Benign naevus
    (d)   Superficial spreading malignant melanoma
    (e)   Squamous cell carcinoma

28. A 21-year-old woman presents with bilateral middle ear effusions. She is generally fit and well except that she is taking medication for panic attacks, which occur when she is in crowded places such as shopping malls. Which of the following drugs is most likely to be responsible?

    (a)   Aspirin
    (b)   Propranolol
    (c)   Phenytoin
    (d)   Rosperidone
    (e)   Frusemide

29. What percentage of longitudinal temporal bone fractures is associated with facial nerve palsy?

   (a)   10%
   (b)   20%
   (c)   40%
   (d)   60%
   (e)   80%

30. The most definitive test for establishing the identification of a foreign body in the upper aerodigestive tract is

   (a)   Contrast swallow
   (b)   PA and lateral neck X-ray
   (c)   AP and lateral neck X-ray
   (d)   Direct endoscopy
   (e)   Lateral decubitus X- ray

31. A 55-year-old woman presents with generalised weakness and bilateral facial nerve palsies. After ruling out raised intracranial pressure, the medical registrar proceeded to a lumbar puncture. The result shows raised CSF protein. What is the most likely diagnosis?

   (a)   Primary Sjogrens
   (b)   Myasthenia gravis
   (c)   Guillain Barre syndrome
   (d)   Melkersson Rosenthal syndrome
   (e)   Moebius syndrome

32. A 40-year-old barmaid presents with a 4 month history of a right throat discomfort. Examination reveals an indurated firm lesion in the right tonsil measuring 3 cm and a lymph node more than 6 cm in greatest dimension in level 2 of the neck. What is the TNM stage?

   (a) T2N1
   (b) T2N2
   (c) T2N3
   (d) T3N2
   (e) T3N3

33. A 24-year-old chocoholic woman presents with a four month history of severe, episodic throbbing left sided headaches associated with tingling in her left hand. The day before each episode she feels unwell and goes off her food, including chocolate. She also describes flashing lights in her left visual field prior to the onset of severe headache. Her headache sometimes last for 72 hours. She describes being asymptomatic between attacks. What is the single most likely cause for her headache?

   (a) Benign (idiopathic) intracranial hypertension
   (b) Cluster headache
   (c) Migraine
   (d) Psychogenic headache
   (e) Space occupying lesion (e.g. brain tumour)

34. Which branchial arch is most commonly involved in the formation of pre-auricular sinuses?

   (a) First
   (b) Second
   (c) Third
   (d) Fourth
   (e) Sixth

35. A 54-year-old woman presents complaining of a dry eyes and mouth. Examination also revealed ulna deviation of her fingers. What is the most likely diagnosis?

   (a)   Relapsing polychondritis
   (b)   Sjögren's syndrome
   (c)   Syphilis
   (d)   Systemic lupus erythematosus
   (e)   Tuberculosis

36. A 10-month-old baby girl presents with difficulty breathing. On examination, she is noted to be obese with significant macroglossia. What is the most likely syndrome in this case?

   (a)   Beckwith-Wiedemann
   (b)   Treacher-Collins
   (c)   Turners
   (d)   Velocardiofacial
   (e)   Jervell-Lange-Neilsen

37. An 18-month-old boy presents with a brief history of choking and cyanosis for about 10 seconds a few hours earlier. He is now completely asymptomatic. What is the likely diagnosis?

   (a)   Acute epiglottitis
   (b)   Chronic obstructive airway disease
   (c)   Allergic reaction
   (d)   Laryngomalacia
   (e)   Foreign body

38.	Which of the following is an indication to adenoidectomy?

(a)	Upper respiratory tract infection
(b)	Obstructive sleep apnoea
(c)	Submucous cleft
(d)	Medially situated internal carotid artery
(e)	Uncontrolled bleeding disorder

39.	A 14-year-old male presents with fever, sore throat, coated tonsils, malaise, wide spread lymphadenopathy and tender abdomen. Which is the most likely infectious disease?

(a)	Cytomegalovirus
(b)	Infectious mononucleosis
(c)	Rubella
(d)	Mumps
(e)	Toxoplasmosis

40.	Which cranial nerve innervates stylopharyngeus?

(a)	Vagus nerve
(b)	Glossopharyngeal nerve
(c)	Facial nerve
(d)	Spinal accessory nerve
(e)	Hypoglossal nerve

41. A 35-year-old female presents with a gradual reduction in hearing on the left side during her pregnancy. There were no other otological symptoms or significant past medical history. On examination she has normal ear canal and tympanic membrane. Weber's lateralizes to the left and Rinne's test is negative. Pure tone audiogram shows a 40dB conductive hearing loss. What is the most likely diagnosis?

    (a) Otitis media with effusion
    (b) Otosclerosis
    (c) Auditory neuropathy
    (d) Noise induced hearing loss
    (e) Presbyacusis

42. A 60-year-old woman presents to her GP with a history of intermittent dizzy sensation lasting between 6-12 hours at a time. This was usually preceded by a feeling of fullness in the ear, together with unilateral hearing loss and tinnitus. What is the most likely diagnosis?

    (a) Migraine
    (b) BPPV
    (c) Menieres disease
    (d) Acute labyrinthitis
    (e) Vertebro-basilar ischaemia

43. A 70 year old man is having sphenopalatine artery ligation when the vessel snap and retract into the pterygopalatine fossa. What is your initial management?

    (a) Pack the nose
    (b) Endoscopic ligation of the maxillary artery via the maxillary antrum
    (c) External carotid artery ligation
    (d) Call a consultant colleague for help
    (e) Arrange for embolization of the maxillary artery.

44. A 52-year-old man presents with a septal perforation. He makes regular overseas business trips. What is the most likely diagnosis?

    (a) Wegener's
    (b) Sarcoidosis
    (c) Relapsing polychondritis
    (d) Syphilis
    (e) Tuberculosis

45. An 84-year-old woman is discovered unconscious at home with a torrential epistaxis and subsequently brought to hospital by ambulance. Arrest of the bleed is required in theatre. Her husband expresses his refusal to allow her to go to theatre. Which of the following statements is the most appropriate next step?

    (a) Make patient ward of court
    (b) Wait for consent from next of kin
    (c) Wait for consent from the patient
    (d) Surgery can proceed
    (e) Surgery cannot proceed

46. Which of the following drug is most likely to cause oral lichenoid reaction as a side effect?

    (a) Ciprofloxacin
    (b) Cisplatin
    (c) Methotrexate
    (d) Augmentin
    (e) Penicillamine

47. CT scan shows ossification of the labyrinthine membrane on the left and MRI does not show the membrane. What is the most likely diagnosis?

    (a) Left labyrinthitis obliterans
    (b) Left Menieres disease
    (c) Left otosclerosis
    (d) Left superior semicircular canal dehiscence
    (e) Left vestibular schwannoma

48. Which of the following statement is TRUE regarding hereditary haemorrhagic telangiectasia?

    (a) Can be effectively treated with a KTP or Argon Laser
    (b) Androgens are effective treatment for both men and women
    (c) Youngs procedure involves excising the septal mucosa and replacing it with a split skin graft
    (d) Malaena is invariably due to ingestion of blood following epistaxis
    (e) Is very rarely life-threatening

49. Juvenile angiofibromas are rare, benign, vascular neoplasms that occur almost exclusively in the nasopharynx of adolescent males. What is the gold standard of treatment?

    (a) Incisional biopsy
    (b) Excision via a mid-facial degloving approach
    (c) Hormone therapy
    (d) Chemotherapy
    (e) Monitoring as will involute with time

50. A 63-year-old woman is admitted under the general surgeons with abdominal pain. She develops bilateral submandibular swellings which is worse on eating. Which is the most appropriate laboratory investigation?

   (a) Full blood count and differential
   (b) Urea and Electrolytes
   (c) ESR
   (d) CRP
   (e) Autoimmune screen

51. LASER is an acronym for light amplication by stimulated emission of radiation. Which would be the most appropriate for removing a tongue lesion?

   (a) Nd:YAG laser
   (b) CO2 laser
   (c) Argon laser
   (d) KTP laser
   (e) Diode laser

52. Deficiency of which coagulation factor is linked to Von Willebrand disease?

   (a) Factor X
   (b) Factor II
   (c) Factor VII
   (d) Factor VIII
   (e) Factor IX

53. Cholesteatoma formation involves retes ridges of the basement membrane. This statement best describes which theory of the aetiopathogenesis of cholesteatoma?

   (a) Acquired inclusion theory
   (b) Amniotic fluid contamination theory
   (c) Basal hyperplasia theory
   (d) Embryonic germ cell distribution theory
   (e) Epidermoid formation theory

54. Jitter in voice pathology represents...

   (a) Pitch period pertubation
   (b) Changes in amplitude
   (c) Changes in resonance of the voice
   (d) The fundamental frequency of the individual
   (e) The power of the voice

55. You are asked to see a 35 yr old man in A&E with left peri-orbital cellulitis and marked proptosis. Repeated clinical examination over a 15 minute period revealed marked deterioration in colour vision and visual acuity. The ophthalmologist on call is in another hospital 50 minutes away and your consultant phone is on voice mail. What is the most appropriate immediate course of action?

   (a) Treat with intravenous steroids, iv mannitol and massage the eye.
   (b) Leave a message on your consultant phone to contact you ASAP
   (c) Await review by the on-call ophthalmologist
   (d) Perform a lateral canthotomy
   (e) Continue to observe until theatre space becomes available

56. Which is the most likely causative virus for Subacute sclerosing panencephalitis?

    (a) Parvovirus
    (b) Rotavirus
    (c) Paramyxovirus
    (d) Astrovirus
    (e) Papovavirus

57. A 24-year-old man presents with pain in his right ear. On examination there is pus in the external ear canal, which appears, erythematous and swollen. What is the most likely diagnosis?

    (a) Cholesteatoma
    (b) Chronic serous otitis media
    (c) Impacted wax
    (d) Otitis externa
    (e) Otitis media

58. Prolonged PR interval,, small T waves and depressed ST segment is associated with which of the following metabolic disorder?

    (a) hypocalcaemia
    (b) hypercalcaemia
    (c) hypokalaemia
    (d) hyperkalaemia
    (e) hyponatraemia

59. What is the commonest ENT manifestation of HIV infection?

(a) Adenoid hypertrophy
(b) Oral candidiasis
(c) Facial nerve palsy
(d) Malignant otitis externa
(e) Parotid cysts

60. What volume of saline is needed to make 1:80,000 solution containing 0.125mg of adrenaline?

(a) 2mls
(b) 4mls
(c) 10mls
(d) 20mls
(e) 40mls

61. A 7-year-old boy presents bilateral hearing loss. Examination reveals down slanting palpebral fissures, microtias, ear canal atresias and bilateral conductive hearing loss. Which branchial pouch is most likely to be responsible?

(a) First branchial pouch
(b) Second branchial pouch
(c) Third branchial pouch
(d) Fourth branchial pouch
(e) Sixth branchial pouch

62. A 52-year-old man present with hearing loss and dizziness when he hears a loud noise such as his alarm clock. Which is the single most likely eponymous name?

    (a) Hitselberger
    (b) Tullio phenomenon
    (c) Gradenigo
    (d) Schwartze
    (e) Bezold

63. A 55-year-old man presents with almost no voice. He was operated on three times for whitish lesions on his vocal folds. Biopsies taken at each operation reveal no evidence of malignancy. What is the most likely diagnosis?

    (a) Chronic laryngitis
    (b) Laryngocoele
    (c) Squamous cell carcinoma of larynx
    (d) Laryngeal papillomatosis
    (e) Keratosis of the vocal folds

64. Which part of the cochlea is damaged by noise induced hearing loss?

    (a) Basal turn
    (b) Stria vascularis
    (c) Apex
    (d) Basilar membrane
    (e) Inner hair cells

65. The variation of weight over a period of 3 months in 600 obese subjects on a calorie controlled weight reducing diet. Which is the most suitable statistical test?

   (a) Kruskal Wallis test
   (b) Mann-Whitney U test
   (c) McNemar
   (d) One Sample (paired) Student's t-test
   (e) One-way analysis of variance (ANOVA)

66. A 75-year-old man present with hearing loss. He is currently receiving cisplatin for a T3N0 laryngeal carcinoma. What is the single most appropriate investigation?

   (a) Urea & electrolytes
   (b) Bone profile
   (c) Blood glucose
   (d) c-ANCA
   (e) p-ANCA

67. What is the most appropriate genetic description for cell division occurring in the germ cell?

   (a) Meiosis
   (b) Mitosis
   (c) Mosaicism
   (d) Trisomy
   (e) Translocation

68. Which cellular mediator is responsible for nasal blockage?

   (a) TNF-α
   (b) IL1
   (c) Complement
   (d) Histamine
   (e) Serotonin

69. Which of the following is not considered a treatment option for achalasia?

   (a) Nifedipine
   (b) Omeprazole
   (c) Botulinum toxin injections
   (d) Oesophageal dilatation
   (e) Myotomy

70. In the mechanism of swallowing, which of the following is not part of the pharyngeal phase?

   (a) Opening of cricopharyngeal sphincter
   (b) Closure of the nasopharynx
   (c) Pushing of the food bolus into the oropharynx
   (d) Lifting of the larynx
   (e) Tightening of the oropharynx by superior constrictor action

71. A newborn baby boy is found to have a large swelling in the anterior neck. It extends retrosternally causing compression and deviation of the trachea with airway compromise requiring immediate intubation and ventilation. An urgent ultrasound scan and FNA reveals a heterogeneous mass, which contains a mixture of undifferentiated and differentiated cells. Which of the following is the most likely cause for the neck mass?

(a) Pilomatrixoma
(b) Thyroglossal cysts
(c) Teratoma
(d) Cystic hygroma
(e) Branchial cyst

72. A 39-year-old woman presents with numbness over the lateral surface of his upper arm 10 days after a neck dissection. Which nerve has most likely been damaged?

(a) C5
(b) C6
(c) C7
(d) C8
(e) T1

73. A 50-year-old woman presents with early morning joint pains, dry eyes and dry mouth. What is the single most likely diagnosis?

(a) Rhomboid glossitis
(b) Cheilitis glandularis
(c) Sialosis
(d) Lichen planus
(e) Sjogrens

74. The geniculate ganglion contains...

   (a) Cell bodies of the chorda tympani
   (b) Cell bodies of the greater superficial petrosal nerve
   (c) Cell bodies of the lesser superficial petrosal nerve
   (d) Cell bodies of Jacobson nerve
   (e) Is known as the hayfever ganglion and found in the sphenopalatine fossa

75. For the chemical composition, Dexamethasone, framycetin and gramicidin, what is the corresponding topical aural preparation?

   (a) Otomize
   (b) Otosporin
   (c) Sofradex
   (d) Betnovate
   (e) Locorten-Vioform

76. A 6-year-old girl presents with suppurative and necrotizing granulomatous lymphadenitis with stellate abscesses. She owns a cat. What is the most likely infective organism?

   (a) Borellia burgdorferi
   (b) Atypical mycobacterium
   (c) Actinomyces
   (d) Rochalimaea (Bartonella) henselae
   (e) Rhinosporidium seeberi

77. All of the following medicines are associated with enlargement of the salivary glands EXCEPT:

   (a) Oral contraceptive Pill
   (b) Carbimazole
   (c) Coproxamol
   (d) Thiouracil
   (e) isoprenaline

78. A 45-year-old man presents with a 4-month history of persistent ear ache and some discomfort on swallowing but no weight loss. He drinks 10 units of alcohol each day for the last 5 years. Examination reveals a 3 cm cancerous ulcer in the left piriform fossa extending from the medial wall to the lateral wall the vocal folds were mobile and symmetrical. Neck examination was normal with no palpable lymph nodes. What is the TNM stage?

   (a) T1N0M0
   (b) T1N1M0
   (c) T1N1aM0
   (d) T1N1bM0
   (e) T2N0M0

79. How much adrenaline is contained in 1 ml of 1:100,000 solution

   (a) 1 microgram
   (b) 10 micrograms
   (c) 100 micrograms
   (d) 1000 micrograms
   (e) 10000 micrograms

80. Which of the following represents an unusual presentation of glomus vagale?

    (a) Pulsatile tinnitus
    (b) Recurrent drop attack
    (c) Facial nerve palsy
    (d) Hypoglossal nerve palsy
    (e) Otalgia

81. With regards lymphatic drainage of the head and neck region; lymph from the tongue drains into which of these nodes before entering the jugular trunk?

    (a) Jugulo-omohyoid nodes
    (b) Jugulo-digastric nodes
    (c) Sublingual nodes
    (d) Submandibular nodes
    (e) Submental nodes

82. A 17-year-old man presents with a thyroid lesion. Fine needle aspiration cytology suggests a non-neoplastic result. Which is the most appropriate Thy staging?

    (a) Thy1
    (b) Thy2
    (c) Thy3
    (d Thy4
    (e) Thy5

83. A 40-year-old man presents with a warty lesion on the nasal septum but no nasal discharge. Which is the most likely diagnosis?

    (a) Cylindrical cell papillomas
    (b) Fungiform papilloma
    (c) Inverted papilloma
    (d) Malignant melanoma
    (e) Lymphoma

84. Pre-ganglionic secretomotor fibres to the submandibular gland are carried in...

    (a) the glossopharyngeal nerve
    (b) the facial nerve
    (c) the lingual nerve
    (d) the hypoglossal nerve
    (e) the trigeminal nerve

85. A 49 year old female lorry driver presents with snoring. A sleep study shows an apnoea-hypopnea index of greater than 30. What would you advise him?

    (a) Continue as before
    (b) Lose weight
    (c) Stop drinking
    (d) Patient to inform DVLA
    (e) Doctor to inform DVLA

86. A 65-year-old female presents with heart failure who complains of daytime somnolence and poor night's sleep. Polysomnography shows apnoea with no thoracic or abdominal movement. What is the most likely diagnosis?

    (a) Periodic limb movement disorder
    (b) Narcolepsy
    (c) Upper airways resistance syndrome
    (d) Central sleep apnoea
    (e) Idiopathic hypersomnolence

87. To assess whether likelihood to pass the state surgery exam is greater in Boston training programme applicants compared to applicants from elsewhere. What is the most suitable statistical test?

    (a) Chi square test
    (b) Spearman's correlation coefficient
    (c) Mann Whitney U test
    (d) Fisher's exact test
    (e) Friedman test

88. A 42-year-old male office worker is noted to have a fistula of the lateral semicircular canal during right tympanomastoid surgery. There is no fluid leak and the defect is filled with bone wax. The patient wakes up feeling dizzy. Weber tuning fork test goes to the right. What type of nystagmus is he likely to have?

    (a) Bidirectional
    (b) Downbeat
    (c) Horizontal to the left
    (d) Horizontal to the right
    (e) No nystagmus

89. Nystagmus produced by pressure applied to a sealed EAC in a patient with syphilic involvement of the otic capsule is known as which sign?

    (a) Griesinger
    (b) Brown
    (c) Hitselberger
    (d) Boyce
    (e) Hennebert

90. A 50-year-old woman presents with severe septicaemia following abdominal surgery. Her BMI is 35 and she requires a tracheostomy for ventilation. The surgeon notes an increased pretracheal space due to excessive amount of adipose tissue. Which is the most appropriate tracheostomy tube?

    (a) Silver negus single lumen
    (b) Adjustable flange tube
    (c) Paediatric tracheostomy tube
    (d) Standard uncuffed non-fenestrated tube
    (e) Standard uncuffed fenestrated tube

91. A 21-year-old man presents with recurrent sinusitis. Investigations reveal situs inversus and immotile cilia. In this case, which of the following syndromes is most likely?

    (a) Cystic fibrosis
    (b) Kartagener's syndrome
    (c) Osler-Weber-Rendu syndrome
    (d) Pierre Robin syndrome
    (e) Young's syndrome

92. A 70-year-old arthritic man from a nursing home complains of hearing loss. His pure tone audiograms reveal bilateral severe sensorineural hearing loss. What is the most appropriate initial hearing device?

    (a) In-the-canal (ITC) hearing aid
    (b) In-the-ear (ITE) hearing aid
    (c) Cochlear implant
    (d) Spectacle CROS hearing aid
    (e) Body-worn hearing aid

93. Which laryngeal muscle is not supplied by the recurrent laryngeal nerve?

    (a) Cricothyroid muscle
    (b) Posterior cricoarytenoid musces
    (c) Lateral cricoarytenoid muscles
    (d) Transverse arytenoid muscle
    (e) Oblique arytenoid muscles

94. The maximum safe dose of which local anaesthetic agent is 3mg/kg without adrenaline.

    (a) Bupivacaine
    (b) Cocaine
    (c) Levobupivacain
    (d) Lignocaine
    (e) Ropivacaine

95. A 4-year-old boy presents for the second time with a unilateral 20 dB conductive hearing loss secondary to otitis media with effusion. His other ear has normal hearing. What is the most appropriate management?

    (a) Repeat hearing test with 6 week time interval
    (b) Repeat hearing test in 3 months
    (c) Recommend hearing aids
    (d) Insert grommets
    (e) Insert grommets and adenoidectomy

96. A 76-year-old man presents with deafness and neuralgia affecting his face on the right side. He is experiencing nasal regurgitation and difficulty in speaking. He has a mass on CT in the nasopharynx. What is the most likely diagnosis?

    (a) Woodruff's plexus
    (b) Tullio's phenomena
    (c) Hennebert
    (d) Melkersson-Rosenthal syndrome
    (e) Trotter's syndrome

97. A 25-year-old woman presents following an assault, opens her eyes spontaneously and is able to localise painful stimuli but mumbles inappropriate words. What is her GCS (Glasgow Coma Score)?

    (a) 10
    (b) 11
    (c) 12
    (d) 13
    (e) 14

98. A 15-year-old girl who had combined approach tympanoplasty 12 months ago for cholesteatoma. The surgeon would like to know if the disease has reoccurred. Which of the following is the most appropriate imaging modality?

   (a) Gadolinium enhanced MRI scan
   (b) MRI non echo planar diffusion weighted
   (c) MRI STIR sequence
   (d) MRI T1 images
   (e) MRI T2 images

99. An 80-year-old man presents with sudden onset in difficulty in swallowing. He lives in a nursing home and was recently diagnosed with dementia. The nurse accompanying him stated that he did not have any previous swallowing problems and had eaten breakfast a few hours ago. What is the most likely diagnosis?

   (a) Vagus nerve palsy
   (b) Stroke
   (c) Oesophageal foreign body
   (d) Oesophageal candidiasis
   (e) Recurrent laryngeal nerve palsy

100. A 65-year-old male presents with recent weight loss describes a blowing tinnitus and echo sensation of his own voice. He admits his symptoms resolve when he has a cold and nasal blockage. Tympanometry shows frequent fluctuations in the trace. What is the most likely diagnosis?

   (a) Stapedius myoclonus
   (b) Palatal myoclonus
   (c) Venous malformation
   (d) Superior semicircular canal dehiscence
   (e) Patulous Eustachian tube

101. A 17-year-old girl presents with lymphadenopathy develops a rash after receiving a prescription from her GP for a sore throat. Which antibiotic therapy would be the most appropriate?

   (a) Oral Penicillin V
   (b) Oral Amoxicillin
   (c) Oral Metronidazole
   (d) Oral Co-Amoxiclav
   (e) Oral Clarithromycin

102. A 40-year-old man presents with dizziness whilst swimming. Two years ago he had a modified radical mastoidectomy for cholesteatoma. The patient requested obliteration of his mastoid cavity to avoid the caloric effect of water whilst swimming. What is the most appropriate biomaterial?

   (a) Surgisis
   (b) Teflon
   (c) Gutta percha
   (d) Hydroxyapatite
   (e) Medpore

103. A 29 year old man presents with evidence of a parapharyngeal space abscess. The most likely microbiological flora responsible for this infection.

   (a) Group A and non-Group A streptococcus
   (b) Anaerobic organisms
   (c) Polymicrobial flora with both aerobic and anaerobic organisms
   (d) Gram-negative organisms
   (e) Staphylococcus aureus

104. A 70-year-old man presents with a soft mass in the tail of his parotid on the left. He is a smoker. FNA shows papillary formations, cystic spaces and a supporting stroma of dense lymphoid tissue with follicles. Which of the following is the most likely diagnosis?

    (a)   Oncocytoma
    (b)   Pleomorphic adenoma
    (c)   Mucoepidermoid carcinoma
    (d)   Sialolithiasis
    (e)   Warthin's tumour

105. Which pharyngeal muscle forms the midline raphe?

    (a)   Superior constrictor
    (b)   Middle constrictor
    (c)   Inferior constrictor
    (d)   Stylopharyngeus muscle
    (e)   Palatoglossus muscle

106. A 25-year-old asthmatic woman presents with severe rhinorrhoea after taking aspirin. What is the most likely diagnosis?

    (a)   Non allergic eosinophilic rhinitis
    (b)   Allergic rhinitis
    (c)   Drug induced rhinitis
    (d)   Idiopathic rhinitis
    (e)   Non allergic occupational rhinitis

107. A 3-year-old boy presents with an offensive unilateral nasal discharge for over 3 weeks. What is the most likely diagnosis?

(a) Nasal polyps
(b) Rhinolith
(c) Foreign body
(d) Mucocoele
(e) Encephalocoele

108. A newborn girl presents with unilateral facial asymmetry and scoliosis. Which of the following is the most likely syndrome?

(a) Cogan's syndrome
(b) Crouzon syndrome
(c) Down's syndrome
(d) Goldenhar syndrome
(e) Pendred's syndrome

109. What is the most appropriate genetic description for the failure of two members of a chromosome pair to separate during meiosis I?

(a) Wild type
(b) Non-disjunction
(c) Translocation
(d) Robertsonian translocation
(e) Trisomy

110. Which lesion is described histologically as having a Swiss cheese pattern?

    (a)   Adenocarcinoma
    (b)   Pleomorphic adenoma
    (c)   Adenoid cystic carcinoma
    (d)   Mucoepidermoid carcinoma
    (e)   Salivary mucocele

111. Which of the following drugs is a weak opioid and a prodrug, possessing weak agonist actions at the μ-opioid receptor, releasing serotonin and inhibiting the reuptake of norepinephrine?

    (a)   Codeine
    (b)   Morphine
    (c)   Oxybutynin
    (d)   Paracetamol
    (e)   Tramadol

112. A 39-year-old Egyptian woman presents with signs and symptoms consistent with infective atrophic rhinitis. What is the most likely pathogen?

    (a)   Streptococcus pneumonia
    (b)   Klebsiella
    (c)   Haemophilus influenza
    (d)   Staphylococcus aureus
    (e)   Pseudomonas aeruginosa

		PAPER THREE
		Answers
1.	B	Goldenhar syndrome
2.	A	Parasympathetic parotid nerve fibres connecting with sympathetic sweat gland fibres using acetylcholine as the neurotransmitter.
3.	D	Mastoid
4.	A	Oxymethazoline spray
5.	A	Selection bias
6.	C	Imbalance
7.	B	Branchial cyst
8.	C	Foramen spinosum
9.	B	Incision lymph node biopsy
10.	E	Vocal cord palsy
11.	D	Pyramidal eminence
12.	D	Thyroid cartilage & arytenoids
13.	D E	Ranula
14.	C	Spine of Henle
15.	D	Mann-Whitney U test
16.	D	Median rhomboid glossitis is best treated with antifungal lozenges
17.	B	Sebaceous cyst
18.	C	Distraction testing
19.	C	Pemphigus
20.	A	Type As
21.	E	No surgery indicated
22.	A	Haller cells
23.	E	Medullary carcinoma
24.	D	HB Grade VI
25.	A	Keratosis obturans

26.	D	60 dB HL
27.	B	Basal cell carcinoma
28.	B	Propranolol
29.	B	20%
30.	D	Direct endoscopy
31.	C	Guillain Barre syndrome
32.	C	T2N3
33.	C	Migraine
34.	A	First
35.	B	Sjogrens
36.	A	Beckwith-Wiedemann
37.	E	Foreign body
38.	B	Obstructive sleep apnoea
39.	B	Infectious mononucleosis
40.	B	Glossopharyngeal
41.	B	Otosclerosis
42.	C	Meniere's disease
43.	A	Pack the nose
44.	D	Syphilis
45.	D	Surgery can proceed
46.	E	Penicillamine
47.	A	Left labyrinthitis obliterans
48.	A	Can be effectively treated with a KTP or Argon Laser
49.	B	Excision via a mid-facial degloving approach
50.	B	Urea and Electrolytes
51.	D	KTP laser
52.	D	Factor VIII
53.	C	Basal hyperplasia theory
54.	A	Pitch period pertubation
55.	D	Perform a lateral canthotomy

56.	C	Paramyxovirus
57.	D	Otitis externa
58.	C	Hypokalaemia
59.	B	Oral candidiasis
60.	C	10mls
61.	D	Fourth branchial pouch
62.	B	Tullio phenomenon
63.	E	Keratosis of the vocal folds
64.	A	Basal turn
65.	D	One sample paired student's t test
66.	A	Urea & electrolytes
67.	A	Meiosis
68.	D	Histamine
69.	B	Omeprazole
70.	C	Pushing the food bolus into the oropharynx
71.	C	Teratoma
72.	A	C5
73.	E	Sjogrens
74.	A	Cell bodies of the chorda tympani
75.	C	Sofradex
76.	D	Rochalimaea (Bartonella) henselae
77.	B	Carbimazole
78.	C	T1N1aM0
79.	B	10 micrograms
80.	C	Facial nerve palsy
81.	A	Jugulo-omohyoid nodes
82.	B	Thy2
83.	B	Fungiform papilloma
84.	B	The facial nerve
85.	D	Patient to inform DVLA
86.	D	Central sleep apnoea

87.	A	Chi square test
88.	D	Horizontal to the right
89.	E	Hennebert
90.	B	Adjustable flange tube
91.	B	Kartagener's syndrome
92.	E	Body worn hearing aid
93.	A	Cricothyroid muscle
94.	D	Lignocaine
95.	B	Repeat hearing test in 3 months
96.	E	Trotter's syndrome
97.	C	12
98.	B	MRI non echo planar diffusion weighted
99.	C	Oesophageal foreign body
100.	E	Patulous Eustachian tube
101.	B	Oral Amoxicillin
102.	D	Hydroxyapatite
103.	C	Polymicrobial flora with both aerobic and anaerobic organisms
104.	E	Warthin's tumour
105.	A	Superior constrictor
106.	C	Drug induced rhinitis
107.	C	Foreign body
108.	D	Goldenhar syndrome
109.	B	Non-disjunction
110.	C	Adenoid cystic carcinoma
111.	E	Tramadol
112.	B	Klebsiella

1. Which is the only tensor muscle of the larynx?

    (a) Cricothyroid muscle
    (b) Posterior cricoarytenoid musces
    (c) Lateral cricoarytenoid muscles
    (d) Transverse arytenoid muscle
    (e) Oblique arytenoid muscles

2. A 65-year-old male alcoholic presents with a 5 day history of a right facial nerve palsy and bruising on the face and body. Examination of his ear revealed purulent discharge obscuring the view of the tympanic membrane. What is the most likely diagnosis?

    (a) Active squamous chronic otitis media
    (b) Bells palsy
    (c) Herpes zoster
    (d) Lyme disease
    (e) Sarcoidosis

3. Which of the following is associated with retinitis pigmentosa?

    (a) Usher syndrome
    (b) Waardenburg syndrome
    (c) Otosclerosis
    (d) Achondroplasia
    (e) Neurofibromatosis

4. What nerve is the submandibular ganglion suspended from?

   (a) lingual nerve
   (b) maxillary nerve
   (c) hypoglossal nerve
   (d) facial nerve
   (e) trigeminal nerve

5. A young woman presents with a history of recurrent white lesions in the oral cavity. They are tender, confluent and self-limiting. What is the most likely diagnosis?

   (a) Lichen planus
   (b) Leukoplakia
   (c) Aphthous ulcers
   (d) Oral thrush
   (e) Acute necrotizing ulcerative gingivitis.

6. Which of the following is NOT a histological type of basal cell carcinoma?

   (a) Nodular
   (b) Cystic
   (c) Morpheaform
   (d) Verrucous
   (e) Keratotic

7. A 35-year-old woman is found to have nystagmus when her head is turned to the right during a Hallpike manoeuvre. What is the most likely type of nystagmus to be present?

   (a) Pendular
   (b) Rotatory geotropic to the left
   (c) Rotatory geotropic to the right
   (d) Upbeat
   (e) Vertical

8. With regards to variant Creutzfeld-Jacob disease (vCJD), which of the following statements is false?

   (a) Is characterised by intracellular vacuolation in neural tissue
   (b) Tonsil biopsy can be used to diagnose vCJD
   (c) Is transmitted through prions proteins
   (d) Standard sterilization techniques do not remove prions from surgical instruments
   (e) Single use instruments increase the risk of vCJD

9. The following are absolute indications for tonsillectomy EXCEPT:

   (a) Recurrent tonsillitis occurring more than 7 times a year
   (b) Suspected tonsillar carcinoma
   (c) Metastatic neck nodes associated with arcinoma of unknown primary
   (d) Severe OSA associated with tonsillar obstruction
   (e) Streptococcus carrier associated associated with endocarditis

10. A 45 year old alcoholic patient presents with gum pains, oral ulcerations and severe halitosis. Physical examination reveals cervical lymphadenopathy, fever, bright red gingiva and marked ulcerative papillae. What is the most likely diagnosis?

   (a) Ludwig's angina
   (b) Vincent's disease
   (c) Lymphoma
   (d) Squamous cell carcinoma
   (e) Severe tonsillitis

11. A 47-year-old woman presents with fever, red eyes, unilateral facial nerve palsy and bilateral enlargements of the parotid glands. Which of the following is the most likely diagnosis?

   (a) Parotid tumour
   (b) Heerfordt's syndrome
   (c) Maffucci syndrome
   (d) Myasthenia gravis
   (e) Multiple sclerosis

12. A 65-year-old smoker presents with a 4 week history of hoarseness and shortness of breath. On examination, his throat is red with white patches. Flexible nasendoscopy revealed a whitish lesion on the right vocal cord but both cords move normally. There was no cervical lymphadenopathy. What is the most likely diagnosis?

   (a) Keratosis of the vocal folds
   (b) Candidiasis of the larynx
   (c) Chronic laryngitis
   (d) Laryngeal papillomatosis
   (e) Squamous cell carcinoma of the larynx

13. All of the following are branches of the facial nerve EXCEPT:

   (a) Temporal
   (b) Posterior auricular nerve
   (c) Lesser superficial petrosal nerve
   (d) Chorda tympani
   (e) Nerve to stapedius muscle

14. Which of the following arteries does not contribute to Kiesselbach plexus?

   (a) Anterior ethmoidal
   (b) Posterior ethmoidal
   (c) Greater palatine
   (d) Sphenopalatine
   (e) Superior labial arteries

15. Which of the following is carcinoma of the oral cavity associated with?

   (a) Sarcoidosis
   (b) Systemic lupus erythematous
   (c) Syphilis
   (d) Macadamia nuts
   (e) Granulomatosis with polyangiitis (GPA) - formerly Wegener's granulomatosis

16. A 50-year-old man presents with oral ulcers after taking sulphonamides. What is the most likely diagnosis?

   (a) Erythema multiforme
   (b) Pemphigoid
   (c) Pemphigus
   (d) Hereditary angio-oedema
   (e) Median Rhomboid glossitis

17. A 5-year-old boy presents with bilateral absence of anti-helicies. Which of the following is the most likely congenital abnormality?

   (a) Microtia
   (b) Canal atresia
   (c) Preauricular sinus
   (d) Submucous cleft
   (e) Bat/prominent ears

18. What anatomical structure is the lateral limit of the epitympanum?

   (a) Facial recess
   (b) Processus cochlearformis
   (c) Prusack's space
   (d) Pyramidal eminence
   (e) Scutum

19. A 36-year-old Chinese male presents with a painless, fluctuant out-pouching of the upper anterior surface of the pinna. He admits he has had multiple minor traumatic insults to this site over the last 3 years. Histology shows dilated lymphatic system within normal tissue planes. Which of the following is the most likely diagnosis?

   (a) Auricular endochondral pseudocyst
   (b) Chondrodermatitis nodularis helicis
   (c) Relapsing polychondritis
   (d) Sebaceous cyst
   (e) Gouty tophi

20. A 28-year-old woman presents with a GP diagnosis of otosclerosis, based on a carhart notch on her pure tone audiogram and a type A tympanogram. Which of the following is the most appropriate diagnostic test?

   (a) Acoustic Reflex
   (b) Auditory Brainstem Response
   (c) Auditory response cradle
   (d) Conditioned response audiometry
   (e) Cortical evoked response audiometry

21. A 29-year-old man presents with a single recurrent blue sessile swelling on the lower lip that ruptures to release viscid salty mucous. What is the single most likely diagnosis?

   (a) Mucocoeles
   (b) Leukoplakia
   (c) Sialosis
   (d) Cheilitis glandularis
   (e) Lichen planus

22. With regards masking in clinical audiology, which rule/ rules refers to air conduction audiometry?

   (a) Rule 1
   (b) Rule 2
   (c) Rule 3
   (d) Rules 1 & 3
   (e) Rules 2 & 3

23. What is the most likely corresponding eponymous name for an air cell related to the sphenoid sinus?

   (a) Haller cells
   (b) Kuhn cells
   (c) Kupffer cells
   (d) Onodi cells
   (e) Schwann cells

24. A 40-year-old woman presents with a steadily enlarging lump at the base of the neck on the right. On examination there is a thyroid nodule with associated lymphadenopathy. She has raised levels of calcitonin on TFTs. What is the most appropriate pathology?

   (a) Graves disease
   (b) Hashimoto's disease
   (c) De Quervain's thyroiditis
   (d) Riedel's thyroiditis
   (e) Endemic goitre

25. A 8 year old child was found to have a Type B tympanogram with a canal volume of 0.9ml. What is the most likely explanation?

   (a) Wax accumulation
   (b) Tympanic membrane perforation
   (c) Otitis media with effusion
   (d) Eustachian tube dysfunction
   (e) Ossicularity

26. With regards the functions and branches of the facial nerve (CN VII):

  (a) Has motor functions only
  (b) Is the main cranial nerve associated with facial sensation
  (c) Gives rise to the lesser petrosal nerve
  (d) Supplies the mucosal glands of the oropharynx
  (e) Give rise to the chorda tympani

27. A 65-year-old female presents with chronic dull unilateral otalgia, otorrhoea and no hearing loss. Examination shows localised erosion postero-inferiorly in external auditory canal. Patient has had myringoplasty 3 years ago. What is the most likely diagnosis?

  (a) Keratosis Obturans
  (b) Necrotizing otitis externa
  (c) Furunclosis
  (d) External auditory canal cholesteatoma
  (e) Squamous cell carcinoma of the external auditory canal

28. A 48-year-old female presents with an exophytic lesion in her nasal vestibule. It bleeds occasionally. What is the most likely diagnosis?

  (a) Basal cell carcinoma
  (b) Benign naevus
  (c) Keloid scar
  (d) Keratoacanthoma
  (e) Papilloma

29. A 45 year old woman swallowed a piece of chicken bone 48 hours ago and is convinced that it is still lodged in her upper throat. She is able to swallow liquids and solids with minimal discomfort. Nothing abnormal is seen on clinical examination, fibre-optic nasendoscopy or lateral soft tissue X-ray of the neck. What is the best course of management?

   (a) Take the patient to theatre for rigid direct pharyngoscopy and oesophagoscopy
   (b) Arrange an urgent CT scan
   (c) Discharge the patient
   (d) Reassure and review the patient
   (e) Arrange an urgent barium swallow

30. A 59-year-old Asian man presents with a history of nasal obstruction and epistaxis. CT scanning shows a mass in the left ethmoid sinus invading the orbit but not the extending intracranially. There are no neck nodes. What is the TNM stage?

   (a) T2N0M0
   (b) T2N1M0
   (c) T3N0M0
   (d) T3N1M0
   (e) T4N1M0

31. A 7-year-old boy presents with upslanting palpebral fissure. Which of the following is the most likely syndrome?

   (a) Down's syndrome
   (b) Goldenhar syndrome
   (c) Pierre-Robin sequence
   (d) Refsum syndrome
   (e) Treacher-Collins syndrome

32. With regards choanal atresia, which is the most common form?

    (a)   Bilateral bony
    (b)   Bilateral membranous
    (c)   Unilateral bony
    (d)   Unilateral membranous
    (e)   Unilateral mixed

33. A 30-year-old man presents with a three month history of severe stabbing right sided headaches centred around the orbit and radiating to the cheek and jaw. The pain wakes him up from his sleep around 2 am every night and he notices nasal blockage and watery eyes. He seeks relief by pacing up and down. The headache goes away after about 40–60 minutes. The headache is not associated with any warning symptoms, visual disturbances or vomiting. What is the single most likely cause for his headache?

    (a)   Tension (myofascial) headache
    (b)   Cluster headache
    (c)   Temperomandibular joint (TMJ) dysfunction
    (d)   Migraine
    (e)   Psychogenic headache

34. Which of the following are major diagnostic criteria for Waardenburg's syndrome?

    (a)   Skin hypopigmentation
    (b)   Heterochronia Iridum
    (c)   Dystopia canthorum
    (d)   Hypoplasia alae nasi
    (e)   Premature graying of hair

35. A 7-year-old girl presents with a history of a hoarse voice for around 4 weeks presents with worsening stridor over the last 72 hours. There is no pyrexia. This has been her third admission in just over a year with a similar problem. What is the likely diagnosis?

   (a) Vocal cord palsy
   (b) Laryngeal papillomatosis
   (c) Laryngomalacia
   (d) Piriform aperture stenosis
   (e) Chronic obstructive airway disease

36. With regards to cleft lip and palate, which of the following statements is true?

   (a) It is more common in girls
   (b) Is more common in the Native American population
   (c) There is no correlation with smoking during pregnancy
   (d) Is not associated with Pierre Robin sequence
   (e) The face and plate are both completely developed at 8 weeks' gestation

37. A 12-year-old female presents with sudden onset of sore throat headache, fever and a scarlet blushing rash that fades with direct pressure. Desquamation occurs after a few days, especially on the feet and hands. Tonsillar inflammation is also present. Which is the most likely infectious disease?

   (a) Erythema infectiosum (slapped cheek disease)
   (b) Hand, foot and mouth disease
   (c) Steven-Johnson syndrome
   (d) Scarlet fever
   (e) Lyme

38. A 55-year-old woman presents with reduced hearing and otalgia in her left ear after spending and an evening in a Jacuzzi. What is the most likely diagnosis?

   (a) Cholesteatoma
   (b) Chronic serous otitis media
   (c) Impacted wax
   (d) Otitis externa
   (e) Otitis media

39. A 23-year-old female presents with difficulty listening to speech, but has no problems with music. She feels her symptomology is worse in the left. Pure tone audiogram is just within normal thresholds. Otoacoustic emissions are present but stapedial reflexes are absent in her left ear. What is the most likely diagnosis?

   (a) Otitis media with effusion
   (b) Otosclerosis
   (c) Auditory neuropathy
   (d) Noise induced hearing loss
   (e) Presbyacusis

40. A 50-year-old man presents with acute onset of a debilitating spinning sensation associated with nausea and vomiting. This occurred shortly after an upper respiratory tract infection, and slowly improved over several days. What is the most likely diagnosis?

   (a) Migraine
   (b) BPPV
   (c) Psychogenic
   (d) Acute labyrinthitis
   (e) Vertebro-basilar ischaemia

41. A 50-year-old male Asian immigrant presents with a significant saddle nose deformity and multiple skin lesions. What is the most likely diagnosis?

    (a) HIV
    (b) Leprosy
    (c) Tuberculosis
    (d) Syphilis
    (e) Systemic lupus erythematosus

42. Which structure is not usually affected by relapsing polychondritis?

    (a) Pinna
    (b) Nasal skeleton
    (c) Cervical spine
    (d) Laryngeal cartilages
    (e) Tracheobronchial tree

43. Electrocochleography done bilaterally shows summating potential to action potential ratio of 0.5 on left and 0.2 on right. What is the most likely diagnosis?

    (a) Left labyrinthitis obliterans
    (b) Left Menieres disease
    (c) Left otosclerosis
    (d) Left superior semicircular canal dehiscence
    (e) Left vestibular schwannoma

44. What malignancy is associated with Sjogren's syndrome?

    (a)   Hodgkin's lymphoma
    (b)   Non-Hodgkin's lymphoma
    (c)   Adenoid cystic carcinoma
    (d)   Accinic cell carcinoma
    (e)   Mucoepidermoid carcinoma

45. A patient is unable to taste bitter, sweet and sour but his sense of smell is intact. Which nerves are most likely to be affected?

    (a)   Chorda tympani, glossopharyngeal and vagus
    (b)   Olfactory, glossopharyngeal and vagus
    (c)   Lingual, glossopharyngeal and vagus
    (d)   Olfactory, chorda tympani and lingual
    (e)   Chorda tympani, lingual and glossopharyngeal

46. A 38-year-old woman presents with a long history of nose bleeds. Nasal examination reveals several red spots on the septal mucosa. The spots were also present on her lips and face. What is the single most likely cause for the nose bleed?

    (a)   Substance Abuse
    (b)   Drug induced
    (c)   Allergic rhinitis
    (d)   Osler-Weber-Rendu disease
    (e)   Granulomatosis with polyangiitis (GPA)   - formerly Wegener's granulomatosis

47. Botulinum toxin has many therapeutic uses. Which of the following conditions is it not used to treat?

   (a) Spasmodic dysphonia
   (b) Temporomandibular joint disorder
   (c) Drooling
   (d) First bite syndrome
   (e) Nasal polyposis

48. All of the following statements are true about Rhinophyma, EXCEPT

   (a) It is a severe form of acne rosacea
   (b) It is associated with chronic alcoholism
   (c) It is more common in Caucasion men than Afrocaribbean men
   (d) It is associated with the organism Demodex follicularis
   (e) It may mask a skin malignancy

49. What is the most appropriate to avoid keloid scarring?

   (a) Large incision
   (b) Only operate on female patients
   (c) No need for concern as hypertrophic scars regress spontaneously
   (d) Plan for secondary procedures to excise scars
   (e) Ensure minimum tension closure

50. Which of the following is not associated with hypercalcaemia?

    (a)   Primary hyperparathyroidism
    (b)   Sarcoidosis
    (c)   Hypothyroidism
    (d)   Thiazide diuretics
    (e)   Acromegaly

51. Which of the following is not true regarding osteoradionecrosis?

    (a)   Hyperbaric oxygen therapy may prevent necrosis
    (b)   There is an increase risk of pathological fractures
    (c)   Pain is a symptom
    (d)   Discharge is a symptom
    (e)   Neutron beam radiotherapy is associated with less radionecrosis

52. A 6 year old girl steps off a merry-go-round after being on it for 6 minutes. She feels dizzy and has nystagmus with fast component to the left. This is due to:

    (a)   Ampullofugal displacement of cupola in left lateral semicircular canal
    (b)   Ampullopetal displacement of cupola in right lateral semicircular canal
    (c)   Ampullofugal displacement of cupola in right posterior semicircular canal
    (d)   Ampullofugal displacement of cupola in right lateral semicircular canal
    (e)   Ampullopetal displacement of cupola in left superior semicircular canal

53. A 6-year-old boy presents with bilateral proptosis, severe headache and loss of sensation over forehead and eyes bilaterally. What is the most likely diagnosis?

    (a) Preseptal cellulitis
    (b) Orbital cellulitis
    (c) Pott's puffy tumour
    (d) Cavernous sinus thrombosis
    (e) Cerebral abscess

54. Which is the most likely causative virus for Croup?

    (a) Herpes simplex virus
    (b) Human papilloma virus
    (c) Parvovirus
    (d) Parainfluenza virus
    (e) Papovavirus

55. A 6-month-old boy presents with mild stridor. Investigations reveal laryngeal chondromalacia and double aortic arches. Which branchial arch is most likely to be responsible?

    (a) First branchial arch
    (b) Second branchial arch
    (c) Third branchial arch
    (d) Fourth branchial arch
    (e) Sixth branchial arch

56. The highest point of the external occipital protuberance. What is the single most likely bony landmark?

   (a) Inion
   (b) Pterion
   (c) Spine of Henle
   (d) Bregma
   (e) Nasion

57. Which one of the following muscles is supplied by C1 fibres hitchhiking along the hypoglossal nerve?

   (a) Anterior belly of digastric
   (b) Posterior belly of digastric
   (c) mylohyoid
   (d) Thyrohyoid
   (e) Cricothyroid

58. All of the following pass through foramen ovale, EXCEPT:

   (a) Mandibular division of trigeminal nerve
   (b) Meningeal branch of the mandibular nerve
   (c) Accessory meningeal artery
   (d) Lesser superficial petrosal nerve
   (e) Emissary vein

59. A 36-year-old female presents with an intermittent strained, strangled breaks in her voice. Her symptoms do not appear during laughing or singing. Which of the following is the most likely diagnosis?

    (a) Spasmodic dysphonia
    (b) Essential tremor
    (c) Reinke's oedema
    (d) Singer's nodules
    (e) Sulcus vocalis

60. Which of the following will increase the power of the study?

    (a) Increasing the number of investigators
    (b) Decreasing the number of investigators
    (c) Increasing the number of participants
    (d) Decreasing the number of participants
    (e) Double-blinding

61. The thyroid gland is derived from which branchial pouches?

    (a) 1st and 2nd pouches
    (b) 2nd and 3rd pouches
    (c) 3rd and 4th pouches
    (d) 4th and 6th pouches
    (e) 2nd, 3rd and 4th pouches

62. With regards to skull base anatomy, where is the trigeminal ganglion found?

    (a) Foramen Ovale
    (b) Infratemporal fossa
    (c) Foramen Rotundum
    (d) Petrotympanic fissure
    (e) Meckels cave

63. A clinician reviews the medical records of all patients who had tonsillectomy over the past 10 years and records the frequency of primary haemorrhage. Follow-up is available for all subjects. The haemorrhage rate is reported using

   (a) prevalence, because the method of data collection is retrospective
   (b) incidence, because the method of collection is prospective
   (c) prevalence because the direction of inquiry is retrospective
   (d) incidence because the direction of inquiry is prospective
   (e) Survival analysis because some observations are censored

64. Which of the following metabolic derangements is associated with shortened QT interval and widened T wave on ECG?

   (a) Hyponatraemia
   (b) Hyperntraemia
   (c) Hyperkalaemia
   (d) Hypocalcaemia
   (e) Hypercalcaemia

65. A 35-year-old woman presents with bruising. She is taking sodium valproate for vertibrobasilar migraine. What is the single most appropriate investigation?

   (a) MPO
   (b) PR3
   (c) Thyroid function tests
   (d) Liver function tests
   (e) Full blood count

66. Which one of the following factors is not commonly associated in the aetiology of Reinke's oedema?

   (a) Male
   (b) Female
   (c) Hypothyroidism
   (d) Smoking
   (e) Reflux

67. Which of the following drugs is an anti-pyretic agent that is hepatotoxic in overdose?

   (a) Paracetamol
   (b) Codeine
   (c) Tramadol
   (d) Diclofenac
   (e) Difflam

68. A 44-year-old housewife presents to her GP complaining of a feeling of a lump in her throat for the past 6 months. She pointed at the level of her thyroid cartilage, but had no pain in her throat. Clinical examination was normal although she was slightly overweight. What is the most likely diagnosis?

   (a) Gastro-oesophageal reflux
   (b) Goitre
   (c) Myasthenia gravis
   (d) Vagus nerve palsy
   (e) Globus pharyngeus

69. A 12-year-old boy presents with a midline neck anomaly, which has a dimple and a hair protruding from it. Which of the following is the most likely cause for the neck mass?

   (a) Teratoma
   (b) Branchial cyst
   (c) Cystic hygroma
   (d) Thyroglossal cyst
   (e) Dermoid cyst

70. The greater petrosal nerve is a branch of which cranial nerve?

   (a) Trigeminal nerve
   (b) Facial nerve
   (c) Glossopharyngeal nerve
   (d) Vagus nerve
   (e) Hypoglossal nerve

71. Comparing average blood pressures between a group of men and women. Which is the most suitable statistical test?

   (a) Pearsons correlation coefficient
   (b) Spearmans rank correlation coefficient
   (c) Two sample (unpaired) Student's t- test
   (d) Two-way analysis of variance (ANOVA)
   (e) Wilcoxon matched pairs test

72. What is the only intrinsic laryngeal muscle outside the larynx?

   (a) Posterior cricoarytenoid
   (b) Lateral cricoarytenoid
   (c) Cricothyroid
   (d) Arytenoid
   (e) Thyroarytenoid

73. The maximum safe dose of which local anaesthetic agent is 1.5mg/kg and duration of action is 30–60 mins.

   (a) Ropivacaine
   (b) Prilocaine
   (c) Cocaine
   (d) Levobupivacaine
   (e) Lignocaine

74. A 78-year-old man presents with an advanced tumour extending beyond the larynx into the trachea. Examination reveals multiple nodes on the left the largest measures 5cm. He also has enlarged nodes on his chest CT. What is the TNM stage?

   (a) T3N1M0
   (b) T3N2M1
   (c) T4N1M0
   (d) T4N2M1
   (e) T4N4M1

75. Which topical preparation contains hydrocortisone, neomycin and polymixin B?

    (a)   Otomize
    (b)   Otosporin
    (c)   Sofradex
    (d)   Betnovate
    (e)   Locorten-Vioform

76. Which of the following is not a side effect of ipratropium bromide?

    (a)   Glaucoma
    (b)   Prostatism
    (c)   Dry mouth
    (d)   Dry eyes
    (e)   Rhinorrhoea

77. Which nerve may be encountered during a laryngectomy procedure as it is related to the greater horn of the hyoid bone?

    (a)   Ansa cervicalis
    (b)   Glossopharyngeal nerve
    (c)   Hypoglossal nerve
    (d)   Lingual nerve
    (e)   Superior laryngeal nerve

78. In rubella, which group of lymph nodes in the head and neck region are most commonly affected?

    (a)   Pre-auricular
    (b)   Post-auricular
    (c)   Submandibular
    (d)   Levels I-III
    (e)   Levels IV-VI

79. What investigation/ investigations are most appropriate for suspected parathyroid hyperplasia?

    (a)   CT scan
    (b)   MRI scan
    (c)   Sestimibi scan
    (d)   Ultrasound and CT scan
    (e)   Ultrasound and Sestimibi scan

80. A 14-year-old boy presents with recurrent epistaxis. Examination reveals a unilateral nasal mass. Which is the most likely diagnosis?

    (a)   Lymphoma
    (b)   Olfactory neuroblastoma
    (c)   Angiofibroma
    (d)   Benign nasal polyps
    (e)   Inverted papilloma

81. What volume of saline is needed to make 1:200,000 solution using 1ml of 1:1000 adrenaline?

    (a)   10mls
    (b)   20mls
    (c)   100mls
    (d)   200mls
    (e)   400mls

82. A 32-year-old female presents with daytime somnolence and poor night's sleep. She describes vivid dreams whilst falling asleep or on awakening. She can fall asleep very easily and without control during the day. Polysomnography shows REM sleep within 5 minutes of sleep. What is the most likely diagnosis?

    (a)   Periodic limb movement disorder
    (b)   Narcolepsy
    (c)   Upper airways resistance syndrome
    (d)   Central sleep apnoea
    (e)   Idiopathic hypersomnolence

83. A 4-year-old male child presents with a right discharging ear, fever and new onset squint in his right eye. Which is the single most likely eponymous name?

    (a)   Boyce
    (b)   Furstenberg
    (c)   Brown
    (d)   Bryce
    (e)   Gradenigo's

84. A 19-year-old female student presents with single-sided sensorineural deafness following a road traffic accident. She is also short sighted and severely needle phobic. What is the most appropriate initial hearing device?

    (a) No device
    (b) Bone anchored hearing aid
    (c) Cochlear implant
    (d) Spectacle CROS hearing aid
    (e) In-the-canal (ITC) hearing aid

85. A 4-year-old Somalian boy presents in casualty with rapid onset of stridor and drooling. He has never been vaccinated. What is the most likely pathogen?

    (a) Streptococcus pneumonia
    (b) Streptococcus milleri
    (c) Haemophilus influenza
    (d) Staphylococcus aureus
    (e) Pseudomonas aeruginosa

86. A 5-year-old girl presents with 40dB conductive hearing loss bilaterally, found after 3 months of watchful waiting. She frequently suffers from upper respiratory tract infections and nasal blockage. What is the most appropriate management?

    (a) Repeat hearing test with 6 week time interval
    (b) Repeat hearing test in 3 months
    (c) Recommend hearing aids
    (d) Insert grommets
    (e) Insert grommets and adenoidectomy

87. A 28 year old woman was assaulted outside a nightclub. You are asked to review her following primary survey as the emergency medicine doctor feels she has isolated facial injuries. On questioning she opens her eyes spontaneously, is able to localise painful stimuli but mumbles inappropriate words. What is her Glasgow Coma Score?

(a) 7
(b) 9
(c) 11
(d) 12
(e) 15

88. A 60-year-old man presents with metastatic neck disease of unknown primary. MRI neck was reported as normal. Which of the following is the most appropriate imaging modality?

(a) Ultrasound
(b) CT scan with contrast
(c) CT scan without contrast
(d) FDG PET CT
(e) MRI STIR sequence

89. What immunoglobulin (antibody) is found in saliva?

(a) IgG
(b) IgE
(c) IgM
(d) IgA
(e) IgD

90. Laser resection of a T1aN0 SCC of the vocal fold involves resection down to which layer?

    (a)   Epithelial layer
    (b)   Superficial lamina propria
    (c)   Intermediate lamina propria
    (d)   Deep lamina propria
    (e)   Vocalis muscle

91. A 17-year-old girl presents with a quinsy and difficulty swallowing. The ENT registrar recommended anaerobic cover in addition to benzylpenicillin. Which antibiotic therapy would be the most appropriate?

    (a)   Oral Metronidazole
    (b)   Oral Clarithromycin
    (c)   IV Cefotaxime
    (d)   IV Co-Amoxiclav
    (e)   IV Metronidazole

92. What Epworth sleepiness score is consistent with moderate Obstructive Sleep Apnoea in adults?

    (a)   0-10
    (b)   11-14
    (c)   15-18
    (d)   19-24
    (e)   >25

93. A 45-year-old man presents complaining of hearing loss. Examination reveals an audibile noise tinnitus which the patient was unaware of. What is the most likely diagnosis?

(a) Superior semicircular canal dehiscence
(b) Patulous Eustachian tube
(c) Carotid stenosis
(d) Spontaneous otoacoustic emissions
(e) Venous malformation

94. Which of the following is the most common tumour of parotid gland?

(a) Pleomorphic adenoma
(b) Warthin's tumour
(c) Mucoepidermoid carcinoma
(d) Adenoid cystic carcinoma
(e) Adenocarcinoma

95. Following removal of an angiofibroma an adult patient was found to have Hb of 8.2 and clinically stable. What is the best management plan?

(a) Observe and repeat FBC
(b) Transfuse 2 units of blood
(c) Start on iron tablets
(d) start on folate tablets
(e) Start on B12 vitamin, iron and folate

96. A 25-year-old woman presents with severe left frontal headache of 2 days duration. She vomited twice in the last hour and now appears drowsy. She is normally fit and well but recently been on a scuba diving holiday. On examination she has neck stiffness and mucopus in both nostrils. What is the most likely infective organism?

    (a)   Actinomyces
    (b)   Bacteroides spp
    (c)   Klebsiella rhinoscleromatis
    (d)   Staphylococci
    (e)   Streptococcus milleri

97. A 25-year-old woman presents with airway obstruction secondary laryngeal trauma sustained in a RTA. She requires a surgical tracheostomy to protect her airway. Which is the most appropriate tracheostomy tube?

    (a)   Silver negus single lumen
    (b)   Uncuffed non-fenestrated
    (c)   Uncuffed fenestrated
    (d)   Cuffed non-fenestrated
    (e)   Cuffed fenestrated

98. A cystic lesion lined by a double layer of epithelium. What is the most likely corresponding lesion?

    (a)   Lymphangioma
    (b)   Salivary mucocele
    (c)   Adenolymphoma (warthins tumour)
    (d)   Adenoid cystic carcinoma
    (e)   Mucoepidermoid carcinoma

99. Topical decongestant, Phenylephrine works on what type of receptors?

   (a) Beta 1
   (b) Beta 2
   (c) Alpha 1
   (d) Alpha 2
   (e) H1

100. A 50-year-old woman presents with nasal crusting and blockage. She is known to have Wegener's granulomatosis. What is the most likely diagnosis?

   (a) Non allergic eosinophilic rhinitis
   (b) Allergic rhinitis
   (c) Drug induced rhinitis
   (d) Idiopathic rhinitis
   (e) Atrophic rhinitis

101. Which of the following statements about Neurofibromatosis type 2 is true?

   (a) Is an autosomal recessive condition
   (b) Is due to mutations in the NF2 gene on chromosome 21
   (c) Leads to development of schwannomas, meningiomas and ependymomas
   (d) Is detected in an offspring of affected parent by the presence of café au lait spots
   (e) Causes sensorineural hearing loss correctable with a cochlear implant

102. What is the most appropriate genetic description for the observed physical characteristics of an individual?

    (a)   Genotype
    (b)   Phenotype
    (c)   Mosaicism
    (d)   Allele
    (e)   Meiosis

103. The digastric muscle receives innervation from which nerve(s)?

    (a)   Trigeminal and vagus
    (b)   Trigeminal and facial
    (c)   Hypoglossal and vagus
    (d)   Hypoglossal and lingual
    (e)   Trigeminal, facial & hypoglossal

104. A 66-year-old man presents with abrupt sensorineural hearing loss in the high frequencies and moderate speech discrimination. What is the single most likely diagnosis?

    (a)   Cogan's syndrome
    (b)   Inner ear condudive presbyacusis
    (c)   Neural presbyacusis
    (d)   Sensory presbyacusis
    (e)   Strial presbyacusis

105. Which clinical feature is not associated with benign nasal polyps?

    (a)   Loss of taste
    (b)   Cosmetic deformity of the nose
    (c)   Epistaxis
    (d)   Headaches
    (e)   None of the above

106. A 25-year-old woman presents with a unilateral conductive hearing loss following pregnancy. Clinical   examination and investigation suggest a diagnosis of otosclerosis. the patient opted for surgery and the   surgeon chose to use a stapes prosthesis that has 'intrinsic memory'. What is the most appropriate biomaterial?

    (a)   Surgisis
    (b)   Teflon
    (c)   Gutta percha
    (d)   Hydroxyapatite
    (e)   Medpore

107. A 25 year old male victim of a house fire presents to A & E. He is alert and communicative with no external burns of the skin is visible. His lips are erythematous with carbonation discolouration around the mouth. No stridor is audible; however, the patient is slightly tachypnoeic and oxygen saturation is 96% with 2 L oxygen. The most appropriate treatment would be

    (a)   Treat the lips with antibiotic ointment, discharge and f/u patient in OPD

    (b)   Administer 100% humidified oxygen and observe for 6 hours.

    (c)   Place a central line for cardiovascular monitoring and admit the patient to ITU

    (d)   Give 100% humified oxygen and admit to ITU

    (e)   Establish a safe airway with a tracheostomy

108. What is the most likely corresponding eponymous name for a neoplastic binucleated cell?

    (a)   Reed-Sternberg cells

    (b)   Russell's bodies

    (c)   Schaumann's bodies

    (d)   Schwann cells

    (e)   Warthin-Finkelday giant cells

109. All of the following statements pertaining to The European Position Paper on Rhinosinusitis and Nasal Polyps 2007 are correct, EXCEPT:

(a) The duration of the disease is divided into acute (less than 12wks) and chronic (greater than 12 weeks).
(b) The severity of the disease is divided into mild (VAS 0-4), moderate(VAS 5-7) & severe (VAS 8-10).
(c) Either nasal blockage or discharge must present to diagnose rhinosinusitis
(d) Mucosal changes within the osteomeatal complex and/or sinuses form part of the clinical definition
(e) Nasal polyps, mucopurulent discharge or oedema forms part of the clinical definition

110. A 39-year-old woman presents with ipsilateral drooping of the eyelid and dilated pupils 2 days after a neck dissection. Which nerve has most likely been damaged?

(a) C6
(b) C7
(c) C8
(d) T1
(e) T1-L2

111. To determine whether air conduction thresholds changes with increasing age. What is the most suitable statistical test?

(a) Pearson correlation coefficient
(b) Spearman's correlation coefficient
(c) Mann Whitney U test
(d) Fisher's exact test
(e) Friedman test

112. Which nerve roots contribute to ansa cervicalis

   (a)   C1 - C2
   (b)   C2 - C3
   (c)   C1 –C3
   (d)   C2 - C4
   (e)   C2 - C5

PAPER FOUR

Answers

1.	A	Cricothyroid muscle
2.	A	Active squamous chronic otitis media
3.	A	Usher syndrome
4.	A	Lingual nerve
5.	C	Apthous ulcers
6.	D	Verrucous
7.	C	Rotatory geotrophic to the right
8.	E	Single use instruments increase the risk of vCJD
9.	A	Recurrent tonsillitis occurring more than 7 times a year
10.	B	Vincent's disease
11.	B	Heerfordt syndrome
12.	E	Squamous cell carcinoma of the larynx
13.	C	Lesser superficial petrosal nerve
14.	B	Posterior ethmoidal
15.	C	Syphilis (5 'S' – smoking spices, spirits, sharp tooth and syphilis)
16.	A	Erythema multiforme
17.	E	Prominent ears
18.	E	Scutum
19.	A	Auricular endochondral pseudocyst
20.	A	Acoustic reflex
21.	A	Mucoceles
22.	D	Rules 1 & 3
23.	D	Onodi cells
24.	B	Hashimoto's disease
25.	C	Otitis media with effusion
26.	E	Give rise to the chorda tympani
27.	D	External auditory canal cholesteatoma

28.	E	Papilloma
29.	D	Reassure and review the patient
30.	C	T3N0M0
31.	A	Down's syndrome
32.	C	Unilateral
33.	B	Cluster headache
34.	B	Heterochronia iridum
35.	B	Laryngeal papillomatosis
36.	B	Is more common in the native American population
37.	D	Scarlet fever
38.	C	Impacted wax
39.	C	Auditory neuropathy
40.	D	Acute labyrinthitis
41.	B	Leprosy
42.	C	Cervical spine
43.	B	Left meniere's diease
44.	B	Non-hodgkin's lymphoma
45.	A	Chorda tympani, glossopharyngeal and vagus
46.	D	Osler-Weber-Rendu
47.	E	Nasal polyposis
48.	B	It is associated with chronic alcoholism
49.	E	Ensure minimum tension closure
50.	C	Hypothyroidism
51.	D	Discharge is a symptom
52.	D	Ampullofugal displacement of cupola in right lateral semicircular canal
53.	D	Cavernous sinus thrombosis
54.	D	Parainfluenza virus
55.	D	Fourth branchial arch
56.	A	Inion

57.	D	Thyrohyoid
58.	B	Meningeal branch of the mandibular nerve
59.	A	Spasmodic dysphonia
60.	C	Increasing the number of participants
61.	C	3rd and 4th pouches
62.	E	Meckel's cave
63.	D	Incidence because the direction of inquiry is prospective
64.	E	Hypercalcaemia
65.	D	Liver function tests
66.	A	Male
67.	A	Paracetamol
68.	E	Globus pharyngeus
69.	E	Dermoid cyst
70.	B	Facial nerve
71.	C	Two sample (unpaired) Student's t-test
72.	C	Cricothyroid
73.	C	Cocaine
74.	D	T4N2M1
75.	B	Otosporin (discontinued in UK May 2014)
76.	E	Rhinorrhoea
77.	C	Hypoglossal nerve
78.	B	Post-auricular
79.	E	Ultrasound and Sestimibi scan
80.	C	Angiofibroma
81.	D	200mls
82.	B	Narcolepsy
83.	E	Gradenigo's
84.	D	Spectacle CROS hearing aid
85.	C	Haemophilus influenza
86.	E	Insert grommets and adenoidectomy

87.	D	12
88.	D	FDG PET CT
89.	D	IgA
90.	C	~~Migration theory~~ Intermediate lamina propria
91.	E	IV Metronidazole
92.	C	15-18
93.	D	Spontaneous otoacoutic emissions
94.	A	Pleomorphic adenoma
95.	A	Observe and repeat FBC
96.	E	Streptococcus milleri
97.	D	Cuffed non-fenestrated
98.	C	Adenolymphoma
99.	C	Alpha 1
100.	E	Atrophic rhinitis
101.	C	Leads to development of schwannoms, meningiomas and ependymomas
102.	B	Phenotype
103.	B	Trigeminal and facial
104.	D	Sensory presbyacusis
105.	C	Epistaxis
106.	B	Teflon
107.	D	Give 100% humified oxygen and admit to ITU
108.	A	Reed-Sternberg cells
109.	B	The severity of the disease is divided into mild (VAS 0-4), moderate(VAS 5-7) & severe (VAS 8-10).
110.	E	T1-L2 *(sympathetic chain)*
111.	B	Spearman's correlation coefficient
112.	C	C1 - C3

1. A bilobed flap is a type of …

    (a)   Advancement flap
    (b)   Rotational flap
    (c)   Transposition flap
    (d)   Interpolated flap
    (e)   Dufourmental flap

2. A 60 year old man presents with an enlarging ulcerative lesion involving the floor of the mouth. Clinical findings that would suggest mandibular invasion include?

    (a)   Tenderness on palpation
    (b)   Pain with eating
    (c)   Decreased sensation along the tongue
    (d)   Decreased sensation along the lower lip
    (e)   Palpable submandibular lymph nodes

3. The best treatment of a 6mm nodular BCC on the forehead is?

    (a)   Radiation
    (b)   Photodymanic therapy
    (c)   MOH micrographic surgery
    (d)   Excision with advancement flap
    (e)   Imiquimoid

4. A 65-year-old man presents with sudden onset of palatal mass that breaks down to produce, painless irregular ulcer complaining of pyrexia and malaise. What is the single most likely diagnosis?

    (a) Apthous ulcer
    (b) Traumatic ulcer
    (c) Necrotizing sialometaplasia
    (d) Subacute necrotizing sialadenitis
    (e) Cheilitis glandularis

5. A 5 year old boy is referred for hearing assessment. Examination reveals downslanting palpebral fissures, depressed cheek bones, deformed pinna and retrognathia. Audiometry reveals a 40 dBHL conductive hearing loss in his left hear. Which syndrome is he most likely to have?

    (a) Down's syndrome
    (b) Treacher Collins syndrome
    (c) Pierre Robin sequence
    (d) CHARGE syndrome
    (e) Goldenhar syndrome

6. A middle age man complains of nasal obstruction after septorhinoplasty. On examination, he has bilateral alar collapse on inspiration. What is the best management plan?

    (a) Cephalic trimming of the lower lateral cartilage
    (b) Caudal trimming of the lower lateral cartilage
    (c) Caudal trimming of the upper lateral cartilage
    (d) Alar batten grafts
    (e) Spreader grafts

7. Following a septorhinoplasty a patient complains of left facial paraesthesia. Which nerve is most likely to be involved?

   (a) Sphenopalatine nerve
   (b) Facial nerve
   (c) Mental nerve
   (d) Palatine nerve
   (e) External nasal nerve

8. A 75-year-old man presents with a unilateral facial nerve weakness associated with ipsilateral ear pain. Examination reveals vesicles in the painful ear. Which is the most likely cause for his facial nerve palsy?

   (a) Ramsay Hunt syndrome
   (b) Lyme disease
   (c) Mononeuritis multiplex
   (d) Guillian-Barre
   (e) Heerfordt

9. A 2-year-old girl presents with a discharge from a congenital opening anterior to the sternomastoid muscle. She is also partially deaf. Which branchial cleft is most likely to be responsible?

   (a) First branchial cleft
   (b) Second branchial cleft
   (c) Third branchial cleft
   (d) Fourth branchial cleft
   (e) Sixth branchial cleft

10. 3-Dimensional cleft between uncinate medially and lamina papyracea laterally. 41 Functional area bounded by middle turbinate medially and uncinate bone laterally. 42. Is formed by the 1st lamella of the lateral nasal wall. What is the most likely corresponding anatomical structure?

   (a) Maxillary sinus ostium
   (b) Anterior osteomeatal unit
   (c) Ethmoid infundibulum
   (d) Uncinate
   (e) Onodi cell

11. The following statements are true about saliva, EXCEPT:

   (a) The sodium content (mmol/L) is lower than that found in blood plasma
   (b) The potassium content (mmol/L) is lower than that found in blood plasma
   (c) The chloride content (mmol/L) is lower than that found in blood plasma
   (d) The calcium content (mmol/L) is similar to that found in blood plasma
   (e) The bicarbonate content (mmol/L) is higher than that found in blood plasma

12. Which of the following is not detrimental following resuscitation?

   (a) hyponatraemia
   (b) hypoxia
   (c) hypothermia
   (d) hypoglycaemia
   (e) hyperkalaemia

13. A patient presents with a 6 months history of a progressive, non-tender, pulsatile mass on the right side of the neck at level 3. Which is the most appropriate diagnostic investigation?

    (a) CT scan with contrast
    (b) CT scan without contrast
    (c) Angiogram
    (d) Ultrasound scan
    (e) MRI/MRA scan

14. Vocal cord granuloma:

    (a) Occurs on the vocal fold
    (b) Involves type IV hypersensitivity reaction
    (c) Are not associated with repeated traumas
    (d) Can arise because of severe acid reflux
    (e) Can be caused by voice therapy

15. Which anatomical area is between the round window niche and the pyramidal eminence?

    (a) Scutum
    (b) Sinus Tympani
    (c) Prussak's space
    (d) Processus cochlearformis
    (e) Tensor Tympani

16. Which branch of the external carotid artery supplies the meninges of the brain?

   (a) Superficial temporal artery
   (b) Maxillary artery
   (c) Posterior auricular artery
   (d) Occipital artery
   (e) Facial artery

17. How many pairs of major salivary glands do we have?

   (a) one
   (b) two
   (c) three
   (d) four
   (e) six

18. A 25-year-old man presents with a single painful white lesion on his gingiva measuring about 2mm in diameter. What is the most likely diagnosis?

   (a) Behcet's disease
   (b) Lichen planus
   (c) Oral candidiasis
   (d) Traumatic ulcer
   (e) Apthous ulcer

19. A 48-year-old woman presents with oral blisters and ulcers. Immunological investigations reveal antibodies to a basement membrane protein. What is the most likely diagnosis?

   (a) Erythema multiforme
   (b) Pemphigoid
   (c) Pemphigus
   (d) Hereditary angio-oedema
   (e) Median Rhomboid glossitis

20. A 5-month-old boy present with failed automated and manual OAE tests. What is the single most appropriate investigation?

   (a) Visual reinforcement audiometry
   (b) Auditory brainstem response
   (c) Pure tone audiometry
   (d) Otoacoustic emissions
   (e) Speech discrimination test

21. What is the most likely corresponding eponymous name for the epithelial nest of cells thought to be the source of congenital cholesteatoma?

   (a) Russell's bodies
   (b) Schaumann's bodies
   (c) Langhan cells
   (d) Michaels's bodies
   (e) Mikulicz's cells

22. A 32-year-old woman presents with a facial nerve palsy and joint pains. She had recently been on a walking holiday in Canada where she developed a flu-like illness associated with a rash. Which is the most likely cause for his facial nerve palsy?

    (a) Bell's palsy
    (b) Lyme disease
    (c) Sarcoidosis
    (d) Myasthenia gravis
    (e) Ramsay Hunt syndrome

23. A 55-year-old woman presents with tiredness that gets worse towards the end of the day. Examination reveals bilateral facial nerve weaknesses associated with bilateral ptosis. What is the most likely diagnosis?

    (a) Primary Sjogrens
    (b) Myasthenia gravis
    (c) Guillain Barre syndrome
    (d) Melkersson Rosenthal syndrome
    (e) Moebius syndrome

24. Which of the following statements pertaining to audiological investigations is INCORRECT?

   (a) Masking for air conduction is necessary if the hearing loss of the test ear is 40dB or more than air conduction in the non-test ear
   (b) A retrocochlear neural type deafness gives a speech discrimination scores far better than those expected from pure tone thresholds
   (c) Masking is essential for bone conduction thresholds when unmasked bone conduction is better by 10 dB or more than air conduction in the test ear
   (d) A carhart's notch is due to ossicular mechanics which transmit bone conducted sound poorly at 2 kHz in the presence of a conductive hearing loss
   (e) Recruitment is an abnormally increased subjective sensation of loudness for a given increase in sound intensity and is characteristic of sensory pathology.

25. A 57-year-old diabetic male presents with one month of unilateral purulent otorrhoea and severe otalgia. Examination shows granulation at bony-cartilaginous junction. What is the most likely diagnosis?

   (a) Furunculosis
   (b) Necrotizing otitis externa
   (c) Keratosis Obturans
   (d) External auditory canal cholesteatoma
   (e) Squamous cell carcinoma of the external auditory canal

26. Evidence obtained from one randomised controlled trial provides what level of evidence?

    (a) Level Ia
    (b) Level Ib
    (c) Level IIa
    (d) Level IIb
    (e) Level III

27. A 48-year-old man presents with congenital blindness and nystagmus. What is the most likely type of nystagmus to be present?

    (a) Upbeat
    (b) Downbeat
    (c) Vertical
    (d) Pendular
    (e) Bidirectional

28. Malignant melanoma should be assessed considering ABCD warning signs, which best describes what these are?

    (a) Asymmetry, Border, Colour, Diameter
    (b) Asymmetry, Burning, Consistency, Discharge
    (c) Asymmetry, Bleeding, Crusting, Distant lesions
    (d) Absence of colour, Bleeding, Consistency, Diameter
    (e) Absence of colour, Border, Crusting, Diameter

29. What is the commonest cause of septal perforation?

    (a) TB
    (b) Sarcoidosis
    (c) Neoplastic
    (d) Cocaine
    (e) Local trauma

30. The following statements are correct in skull base fracture involving the temporal bone, EXCEPT:

(a) Sensorineural deafness with a pneumolabyrinth on CT scanning is reversible
(b) Longitudinal fractures are commoner than transverse and usually causes conductive deafness
(c) Transverse fractures more commonly cause facial paralysis than longitudinal fractures
(d) Ecchymosis over the mastoid is a common sign
(e) Haemotympanum presents with a blue/black eardrum.

31. A 40-year-old barmaid presents with a 4 month history of a right throat discomfort. Examination reveals an indurated firm lesion in the right tonsil measuring 1.5cm and a 2.5 cm ipsilateral solitary lymph node in level 2 of the neck.   What is the TNM stage?

(a) T1N1
(b) T1N2
(c) T2N1
(d) T2N2
(e) T3N3

32. A 34-year-old woman presents to clinic with a three month history of headache. It tends to occur when she is supine and is worse in the mornings. The headache is exacerbated by coughing, straining and bending over. She also complains of several episodes of transient blurring of vision. Examination reveals an obese female with mild bilateral papilloedema. She has no other neurological signs. What is the single most likely cause for her headache?

    (a) Space occupying lesion (e.g. brain tumour)
    (b) Cerebrovascular accident
    (c) Cluster headache
    (d) Cervical Spondylosis
    (e) Benign (idiopathic) intracranial hypertension

33. A 1-year-old boy presents with expiratory stridor. There was no history of foreign body inhalation or asthma. Microlaryngoscopy and bronchoscopy reveals a partial obstruction within the lumen of the trachea. Which of the following is the most likely congenital abnormality?

    (a) Cleft palate
    (b) Submucous cleft
    (c) Tracheal stenosis
    (d) Tracheal web
    (e) Tracheomalacia

34. Which cranial nerve is found in the pterygopalatine fossa?

    (a) Ophthalmic nerve (V1)
    (b) Maxillary nerve (V2)
    (c) Mandibular nerve (V3)
    (d) Facial nerve
    (e) Glossopharyngeal nerve

35. A 3month old baby boy presents with mild inspiratory stridor. He is growing well and has no developmental delay. Flexible nasendoscopic examination in the clinic reveals posterior laryngomalacia. What is the best management plan?

    (a) Reassure and discharge
    (b) Microlaryngoscopy and bronchoscopy to confirm diagnosis
    (c) Prednisolone to encourage cartilage maturation
    (d) Regular assessment of weight and height
    (e) Regular laryngoscopy to access progress

36. A 21-year-old man presents with sudden onset of conjunctival, nasal, genital lesions, and exfoliating lesions on the hand and feet, following sulphonamide therapy. Which is the most likely infectious disease?

    (a) Hand, foot and mouth disease
    (b) Steven-Johnson syndrome
    (c) Scarlet fever
    (d) Rubella
    (e) Kawasaki

37. MRI scan confirms the diagnosis of a left vestibular schwannoma in a patient. Which of the following clinical features is most common?

    (a) Facial weakness
    (b) Tinnitus
    (c) Bilateral sensorineural hearing loss
    (d) Vertigo
    (e) Diplopia

38. A 4-year-old boy presents with normal hearing at birth who has had a stepwise deterioration in bilateral sensorineural hearing. He is found to be hypothyroid and has a goitre. What is the most likely diagnosis?

    (a) Menieres disease
    (b) Waadenburg syndrome type I
    (c) Waardenburg syndrome type IV
    (d) Pendred syndrome
    (e) Presbyacusis

39. Which bone is situated posterior to the maxillary ostium?

    (a) Lacrimal
    (b) Maxilla
    (c) Palatine
    (d) Uncinate
    (e) Inferior turbinate

40. The Mustarde technique used in otoplasty

    (a) Decreases the cupping and displacement of the pinna by placing chondral mastoid sutures
    (b) Recreates the antihelix by incorporating permanent scapha chonchal and scapha fossa triangularis horizontal mattress sutures
    (c) Recreates the antihelix by incising the cartilage and placing buried mattress sutures
    (d) Involves making parallel cartilage incisions to weaken the cartilage
    (e) Involves scoring the anterior aspect of the auricular cartilage to create posterior bending

41. Pure tone audiogram shows left conductive hearing loss. Tympanometry is normal and ear examination reveals no abnormality. What is the most likely diagnosis?

    (a) Labyrinthitis obliterans
    (b) Menieres disease
    (c) Otosclerosis
    (d) Superior semicircular canal dehiscence
    (e) Vestibular schwannoma

42. A 45-year-old Caucasian female presents with a sudden onset of unilateral otalgia and erythema over right pinna. Has occurred once before but was self resolving within 2 weeks. May have had trauma but cannot remember. Swelling of whole pinna sparing the lobule. Histology shows infiltration of T lymphocytes. Which of the following is the most likely diagnosis?

    (a) Chondrodermatitis nodularis helicis
    (b) Gouty tophi
    (c) Pinna cellulitis
    (d) Relapsing polychondritis
    (e) Telephone ear

43. Which of the following nerve/ nerves is not at risk during submandibular gland excision?

    (a) Marginal mandibular nerve
    (b) Glossopharyngeal nerve
    (c) Hypoglossal nerve
    (d) Lingual nerve
    (e) None of the above – all 4 nerves are at risk

44. Which vasculitic disease is characterised by a prodromal stage of allergic rhinitis, nasal polyposis and asthma?

   (a) Polyarteritis nodosa
   (b) Wegener's granulomatosis
   (c) Churg-Strauss
   (d) Sarcoidosis
   (e) Bechet

45. With regards to diathermy, which one option is true?

   (a) Uses D.C. current through body tissues
   (b) Uses electrical frequency from 300kHz to 3 MHz
   (c) Uses electrical frequency at 50kHz
   (d) Uses temperatures of 100 degrees Celsius
   (e) Is measured in Joules

46. A 2-year-old boy presents with a blood-stained foul smelling mucopurulent discharge from one nostril. Examination reveals inflamed mucous membrane. What is the single most likely cause for the nose bleed?

   (a) Iatrogenic
   (b) Foreign body
   (c) Rhinolith
   (d) Pyogenic granuloma
   (e) Juvenile angiofibroma

47. A 40-year-old female presents to clinic complaining of a change in her sense of smell. What is a well-validated and reliable test you could arrange?

    (a) University of Bristol Sniff test
    (b) University of Pennsylvania Smell Identification Test
    (c) Taste and Smell Clinic Vinegar test
    (d) Threshold olfactory test
    (e) Positive Smell Test

48. Which of the following statements about the nasal cavity is true?

    (a) Main blood supply is from the nasociliary artery
    (b) Heavy epistaxis related to nasal fractures is due to damage to the sphenopalatine artery
    (c) The veins have no valves
    (d) Parasympathetic nerve supply is derived from the trigeminal nerve
    (e) The vomer is attached to the cribiform plate

49. How many types of paraganglioma affect the head and neck region?

    (a) 2
    (b) 3
    (c) 4
    (d) 5
    (e) 6

50. Which of the following statements regarding benign fibro-osseous disease is true?

   (a) Cortical bone is replaced with elastic connective tissue
   (b) Is caused by constitutional activation of the G-protein
   (c) Mono-ostotic can be related to McCune-Albright syndrome
   (d) Is more common in females
   (e) Normally stops growing after puberty

51. Your are a member of the interview panel for higher surgical trainee appointments. Each panel member gets to ask one question. Which question would you consider most INAPPROPRIATE?

   (a) Do you plan to take study leave to attend a course?
   (b) Do you plan to utilise your full 2 weeks of paternity leave?
   (c) Do you need any time off between 9-5pm during the week for religious purposes?
   (d) Will you be taking time off if your child is ill?
   (e) Do you plan to utilise your full study leave entitlement?

52. A 6-year-old boy presents with a painful doughy swelling on his forehead following acute sinusitis. What is the most likely diagnosis?
   (a) Preseptal cellulitis
   (b) Orbital cellulitis
   (c) Pott's puffy tumour
   (d) Cavernous sinus thrombosis
   (e) Cerebral abscess

53. Which is the most likely causative virus for infectious mononucleosis?

   (a) Cyclomegalovirus
   (b) Hepatitis C virus
   (c) Parainfluenza virus
   (d) Herpes zoster virus
   (e) Epstein Barr Virus

54. In recurrent respiratory papillomatosis biology, which of the following is considered the most aggressive?

   (a) HPV 6
   (b) HPV 11
   (c) HPV 16
   (d) HPV 18
   (e) HPV 22

55. A 5-year-old boy presents with cleft palate and glue ear, proven over multiple time points and resulting in 40dB conductive hearing loss. What is the most appropriate management?

   (a) Repeat hearing test with 6 week time interval
   (b) Repeat hearing test in 3 months
   (c) Recommend hearing aids
   (d) Insert grommets
   (e) Insert grommets and adenoidectomy

56. A 27-year-old pregnant smoker presents complaining of nasal blockage and rhinorrhoea. What is the most likely diagnosis?

    (a)   Atrophic rhinitis
    (b)   Allergic rhinitis
    (c)   Drug induced rhinitis
    (d)   Hormonal rhinitis
    (e)   Non allergic occupational rhinitis

57. A newborn baby presents with stridor and feeding difficulties. Microlaryngoscopy and bronchoscopy reveal subglottic narrowing secondary to undevelopment of the cricoid cartilage. Which branchial abnormality can explain this defect?

    (a)   First branchial apparatus
    (b)   Second branchial aparatus
    (c)   Third branchial apparatus
    (d)   Fourth branchial apparatus
    (e)   Sixth branchial apparatus

58. Which skull base foramen is the entry port of the spinal division of the accessory into the cranium?

    (a)   Foramen Magnum
    (b)   Jugular foramen
    (c)   Hypoglossal foramen
    (d)   Petrotympanic fissure
    (e)   Stylomastoid foramen

59. Vidian canal opens into which fossa?

    (a)   Infratemporal fossa
    (b)   Pterygopalatine fossa
    (c)   Sphenoid fossa
    (d)   Pyriform sinus
    (e)   Supraclavicular fossa

60. What is the recommended resection margin for a 3mm cutaneous malignant melanoma?

    (a)   1cm
    (b)   2cm
    (c)   3cm
    (d)   4cm
    (e)   5cm

61. A 39-year-old woman presents four weeks following an operation on the neck was unable to flex the metacarpophalangeal joints. There also appears to be wasting of the dorsal interossei muscles. Which nerve has most likely been damaged?

    (a)   C6
    (b)   C7
    (c)   C8
    (d)   T1
    (e)   T1-L2 (sympathetic chain)

62. A 45-year-old man presents following a road traffic accident. Within 48 hours of the accident, he complains of severe headache and passing excessive amounts of urine. What is the single most appropriate investigation?

    (a)   Urea & electrolytes
    (b)   Serum and urine osmolality
    (c)   Bone profile
    (d)   Liver function tests
    (e)   Blood glucose

63. A 5 year old boy presents with suspected allergic rhinitis. He has a positive family history of allergy. Which blood test would be most helpful to confirm the diagnosis?

    (a)   Full blood count
    (b)   IgA
    (c)   IgG
    (d)   IgE
    (e)   IgM

64. What is the distance from incisor to cricopharyngeus?

    (a)   15cm
    (b)   20cm
    (c)   25cm
    (d)   30cm
    (e)   35cm

65. A 23-year-old male drug addict presents to Accident and Emergency with a history of pain and difficulty in swallowing over the past week. He had a chronic cough and weight loss, and had been treated previously in the department for abscesses at the injection sites. What is the most likely diagnosis?

    (a) Oesophageal foreign body
    (b) Pharyngeal pouch
    (c) Gastro-oesophageal reflux
    (d) Oesophageal candidiasis
    (e) Stroke

66. A new screening for a lethal disease is going to be introduced in the whole population. The prevalence of the disease is 0.5 percent. The screening process has a risk of carcinogenesis of 1 in 4million. Which statement do you consider most important?

    (a) The sensitivity of the screening test is 97%
    (b) The specificity of the screening test is 97%
    (c) The treatment of early detected disease improves the cure rate in 75% of the patients
    (d) The cost of each screening test is 35p
    (e) The condition affects only a population of over 75 years old.

67. What is the shortest of the cranial nerves and is also capable of regeneration?

    (a) Olfactory nerve
    (b) Audiovestibular nerve
    (c) Abducens nerve
    (d) Occulomotor nerve
    (e) Trochlear nerve

68. In carrying out a facelift procedure to tighten the skin of the face and neck, which of the following is NOT true?

   (a) Injury to the great auricular nerve can be prevented by raising the flap superficial to the sternocleidomastoid fascia
   (b) Injury to the great auricular nerve most commonly occurs where it crosses the sternocleidomastoid muscle
   (c) The face-lift is a rotation advancement flap
   (d) The marginal mandibular branch of the facial nerve may be damaged by dissection just superficial to the platysma muscle
   (e) The marginal mandibular branch of the facial nerve may be damaged by extended sub SMAS (superficial musculoaponeurotic system)

69. Which of the following is not a recognized landmark for identifying the facial nerve?

   (a) Base of the styloid process
   (b) The stylomastoid suture
   (c) The petrotympanic fissure
   (d) Digastric muscle
   (e) Tragal pointer

70. What is the amount of lidocaine present in 100 ul (ie 1 puff) of Co-phenylcaine which contains 5% lidocaine?

   (a) 5mcg
   (b) 10mg
   (c) 1mg
   (d) 50mg
   (e) 5mg

71. Which of the following drugs is associated with Reye's syndrome in children?

    (a) Paracetamol
    (b) Codeine
    (c) Aspirin
    (d) Diclofenac
    (e) Tramadol

72. Which neck level contains upper jugular lymph nodes?

    (a) Level I
    (b) Level II
    (c) Level III
    (d) Level IV
    (e) Level VI

73. For the chemical composition, Dexamethasone, neomycin and acetic acid, what is the corresponding topical aural preparation?

    (a) Otomize
    (b) Otosporin
    (c) Sofradex
    (d) Betnovate
    (e) Locorton-Vioform

74. A 6-month-old boy presents with poor suckling reflex. On examination he was noted to have bilateral squints and facial nerve palsies, which was present since birth. He was born at 40 weeks' gestation by forceps delivery. Which of the following is the most likely diagnosis?

  (a) Guillain Barre syndrome
  (b) Heerfordt's syndrome
  (c) Maffucci syndrome
  (d) Melkersson-Rosenthal syndrome
  (e) Moebius syndrome

75. Multiple endocrine neoplasia is associated with what form of thyroid carcinoma?

  (a) Anaplastic thyroid carcinoma
  (b) Medullary thyroid carcinoma
  (c) Follicular thyroid carcinoma
  (d) Papillomatous thyroid carcinoma
  (e) Lymphoma

76. A 14-year-old boy presents with unilateral nasal obstruction. A CT scan reveals a unilateral homogenous maxillary mass with destruction of the adjacent bone. Which is the most likely diagnosis?

  (a) Angiofibroma
  (b) Mucoepidermoid carcinoma
  (c) Olfactory neuroblastoma
  (d) Rhabdomyosarcoma
  (e) Inverted papillomas

77. A 4-year-old female presents with nasal blockage, snoring and witnessed episodes of obstructive sleep apnoea. She is irritable in the morning and has poor concentration throughout the day. What is the most appropriate treatment?

   (a) Tonsillectomy
   (b) Adenoidectomy
   (c) Adenotonsillectomy
   (d) SMD inferior turbinates
   (e) No surgery indicated

78. A common finding in patients with OSA is?

   (a) Clubbing of nails
   (b) psychosis
   (c) hypertension
   (d) narcolepsy
   (e) nasal obstruction

79. What sign is associated with temporal bone fractures?

   (a) Bocca's sign
   (b) Battle's sign
   (c) Stankiewick's sign
   (d) Hitselberger's sign
   (e) Aquino's sign

80. A 45-year-old man presents with a 6months history of a neck lump. Examination reveals a nodule in the right thyroid lobe and a 2 cm level 5 lymph node. Ultrasound scan revealed a 2cm lesion in the thyroid gland and FNAC suggests papillary carcinoma. What is the most appropriate TNM stage?

   (a) T1N0M0
   (b) T1N1M0
   (c) T1N1aM0
   (d) T1N1bM0
   (e) T2N0M0

81. A 12-year old girl presents with a bifid uvula. Which of the following is the most likely congenital abnormality?

   (a) Cleft palate
   (b) Submucous cleft
   (c) Tracheal stenosis
   (d) Tracheomalacia
   (e) Choanal atresia

82. After acoustic neuroma surgery, what would be the most appropriate option for rehabilitation of hearing loss?

   (a) Small in the ear hearing aids
   (b) Contralateral routing of signal
   (c) Bone anchored hearing aid
   (d) Cochlear implant
   (e) Brainstem implant

83. A 55-year-old woman presents with spontaneous CSF rhinorrhoea. Her BMI is 38. Which of the following is the most appropriate imaging modality?

    (a) X-Ray
    (b) CT scan with contrast
    (c) CT scan without contrast
    (d) MRI T1 images
    (e) MRI T2 images

84. Which structure lies immediately medial to the facial recess?

    (a) Sinus tympani
    (b) Facial nerve
    (c) Chorda tympani
    (d) Pyramidal process
    (e) Stapes

85. A 3 week old baby presents with a rapidly enlarging right parotid swelling. On examination, it is soft and the skin above appears normal. Haematological profile is normal except for a mildly reduced platelet count. What is the most likely diagnosis?

    (a) Mumps
    (b) Rhabomyosarcoma
    (c) Pleomorphic adenoma
    (d) Enlarged lymph node
    (e) Haemangioma

86. A 45-year-old man presents complaining of pulsatile noise in his left ear. The noise decreases when he performs a valsalva manoeuvre. What is the most likely diagnosis?

    (a) Venous malformation
    (b) Superior semicircular canal dehiscence
    (c) Patulous Eustachian tube
    (d) Dural arterio-venous fistula
    (e) Carotid stenosis

87. A 4-year-old boy presents with epiglottitis. Which antibiotic therapy would be the most appropriate?

    (a) Oral Penicillin V
    (b) Oral Erythromycin
    (c) IV Benzylpenicillin
    (d) IV Co-Amoxiclav
    (e) IV Cefotaxime

88. Which of the following suture materials would be best to repair vascular injury during neck dissection?

    (a) PDS
    (b) Silk
    (c) Nylon
    (d) 6/0 Prolene
    (e) Vicryl

89. MRI scan cannot be performed in patients with which devices?

    (a)   (CROS) contralateral routing of signal
    (b)   Behind the ear hearing aid
    (c)   In the canal hearing aid
    (d)   Bone anchored hearing aid
    (e)   Cochlear implant

90. A 45-year-old male Mexican presents with mucopurulent rhinorrhoea. Examination reveals inflamed nasal mucosa and intranasal nodules. What is the most likely infective organism?

    (a)   Psuedomonas aeruginosa
    (b)   Bacteroides spp
    (c)   Klebsiella rhinoscleromatis
    (d)   Staphylococci
    (e)   Streptococcus milleri

91. Approximately what percentage of patient's suffer from Frey's syndrome following parotid surgery?

    (a)   1%
    (b)   10%
    (c)   <50%
    (d)   >50%
    (e)   100%

92. Benign lesion containing foci of mucus, hyaline and cartilage. What is the most likely corresponding lesion?

    (a) Adenocarcinoma
    (b) Pleomorphic adenoma
    (c) Adenoid cystic carcinoma
    (d) Mucoepidermoid carcinoma
    (e) Salivary mucocele

93. Vasomotor or Autonomic rhinitis is often treated with ipratropium bromide. This agent works by

    (a) Acting as a topical anticholinergic and inhibiting mucosal glandular secretion of the nasal cavity
    (b) Decreasing mucosal inflammation in the nasal cavity
    (c) Inducing atrophic changes to the nasal mucosa
    (d) vasoconstriction
    (e) vasodilation

94. Which intracellular component is the site of synthesis of secretory proteins?

    (a) Rough endoplasmic reticulum
    (b) Smooth endoplasmic reticulum
    (c) Golgi apparatus
    (d) Microtubules
    (e) Mitochondria

95. A 70-year-old woman presents with bilateral symmetric sensorineural loss with an upward slope toward the high frequencies and preserved speech discrimination. What is the single most likely diagnosis?

   (a) Cogan's syndrome
   (b) Inner ear conductive presbyacusis
   (c) Neural presbyacusis
   (d) Sensory presbyacusis
   (e) Strial presbyacusis

96. A 12-year-old girl presents with bilateral profound sensorineural hearing following meningitis and requires bilateral cochlear implants. The father is a biomaterial engineer and would like to know about the material used to make the cochlear implant electrode. What is the most appropriate biomaterial?

   (a) Teflon
   (b) Copper
   (c) Titanium
   (d) Platinum
   (e) Stainless steel

97. Which of the following statements about the basal lamella of the paranasal sinuses is INCORRECT?

   (a) The inferior turbinate is one of the lamellae
   (b) The middle turbinate is one of the lamellae
   (c) The sinus lateralis is between the second and third lamella
   (d) The anterior ethmoid artery can be found between the second and third lamella close to the skull base
   (e) The uncinate process is one of the lamella

98. A 17-year-old man is involved in a road traffic accident. He has no response to commands and only extends his arm to pain. His eyes remain closed. What is his GCS (Glasgow Coma Score)?

   (a)   1
   (b)   2
   (c)   3
   (d)   4
   (e)   5

99. To assess nasal outflow, which is the most appropriate test that can be performed in the Office setting?

   (a)   Manometric rhinometry
   (b)   Nasal expiratory peak flow
   (c)   Rhinomanometry
   (d)   Rhinostereometry
   (e)   Spatula misting

100. According to ARIA guidelines, the best treatment for itching associated with allergic rhinosinusitis is?

   (a)   Steroid spray
   (b)   Oral steroids
   (c)   Anti-histamines
   (d)   Saline douch
   (e)   Erythromycin

101. A 10-year-old Greek boy presents for genetic screening because of a suspected clotting disorder. The result reveals a common X-linked single gene disorder that affects clotting. What is the most likely genetic condition?

    (a)   Klinefelter syndrome
    (b)   Thalassaemia trait
    (c)   Haemophila A
    (d)   Prader-Willi syndrome
    (e)   Osteogenesis imperfecta

102. A 5-year-old boy presents with suspicion of a hearing loss. What is the single most appropriate investigation?

    (a)   Visual reinforcement audiometry
    (b)   Auditory brainstem response
    (c)   Pure tone audiometry
    (d)   Otoacoustic emissions
    (e)   Speech discrimination test

103. A 60-year-old man presents with 4-day-old tracheostomy tube in situ. He now requires upper airway airflow in order for him to speak. Which is the most appropriate tracheostomy tube?

    (a)   Uncuffed fenestrated
    (b)   Cuffed fenestrated
    (c)   Cuffed non-fenestrated
    (d)   Uncuffed non-fenestrated
    (e)   Silver negus single lumen

104. A patient presents 3 days after FESS complaining of clear rhinorhoea, especially when he leans forward. What is your next management step?

    (a)   Admit for iv antibiotics
    (b)   Admit for bed rest and lumber puncture
    (c)   Send sample for B2 transferrin analysis
    (d)   Perform halo test
    (e)   Take patient to theatre for endoscopic repair.

105. What are causative factors associated with Barrett's oesophagus?

    (a)   Gastro-oesophageal reflux disease
    (b)   Blood group A
    (c)   Excess Alcohol intake
    (d)   Osler-Weber-Rendu
    (e)   Helicobacter pylori infection

106. Correlation of the blood pressure and age between a group of men and women. What is the most suitable statistical test?

    (a)   Pearson correlation coefficient
    (b)   Spearman's correlation coefficient
    (c)   Mann Whitney U test
    (d)   Fisher's exact test
    (e)   Friedman test

107. A 78-year-old woman presents with a watery eye. Lacrimal syringing of the lower punctum shows reflux from the upper punctum but no penetration into the nose. What is the most likely diagnosis?

    (a)   Canalicular stenosis
    (b)   Conjunctival disease
    (c)   Extropion
    (d)   Nasolacrimal duct blockage
    (e)   Punctual stenosis

108. A 57 year old patient who is severely deaf from left mastoid surgery presents with a 3.7cm left acoustic neuroma. The other ear has satisfactory hearing. Which of the following is the optimal approach to treatment?

    (a)   Medial fossa approach
    (b)   Posterior fossa approach
    (c)   Translabyrinthine approach without brainstem implant
    (d)   Translabyrinthine approach with brainstem implant
    (e)   Stereotactic radiosurgery

109. What is the main pathogen associated with tonsillitis?

    (a)   Staphylococcus
    (b)   Streptococcal
    (c)   Klebsiella
    (d)   Diptheria
    (e)   Epstein Barr Virus

110. Which of the following arteries is a branch of the ophthalmic artery?

    (a)   Anterior ethmoidal
    (b)   Internal maxillary artery
    (c)   Greater palatine
    (d)   Sphenopalatine
    (e)   Superior labial arteries

111. What is the usual age range for which patients with Ménière's disease present?

    (a)   <20 yrs
    (b)   20-40 yrs
    (c)   40-60 yrs
    (d)   60-80 yrs
    (e)   >80 years

112 What is the chemical constituent in Avamys?

    (a)   Iodoform, benzoin & storax
    (b)   Iodoform Paraffin Bismuth
    (c)   Fluticasone fuorate
    (d)   Fluticasone proprionate
    (e)   Ipratropium bromide

		PAPER FIVE
		Answers
1.	C	Transposition flap
2.	D	Decreased sensation along the lower lip
3.	D	Excision with advancement flap
4.	C	Necrotizing sialometaplasia
5.	B	Treacher Collins syndrome
6.	D	Alar batten grafts
7.	E	External nasal nerve
8.	A	Ramsay Hunt syndrome
9.	B	Second branchial cleft
10.	C	Ethmoid infundibulum
11.	B	The potassium content (mmol/L) is lower than that found in blood plasma
12.	C	hypothermia
13.	E	MRI / MRA scan
14.	D	Can arise because of severe acid reflux
15.	B	Sinus tympani
16.	B	Maxillary artery
17.	C	3
18.	E	Apthous ulcer
19.	B	Pemphigoid
20.	B	Auditory brainstem response
21.	D	Michael's bodies
22.	B	Lyme disease
23.	B	Myasthenia gravis
24.	B	A retrocochlear neural type deafness gives a speech discrimination scores far better than those expected from pure tone thresholds
25.	B	Necrotizing otitis externa
26.	B	Level IB

27.	D	Pendular
28.	A	Asymmetry, border, colour, diameter
29.	E	Local trauma
30.	A	Sensorineural deafness with a pneumolabyrinth on CT scanning is reversible
31.	A	T1N1
32.	E	Benign (idiopathic) intracranial hypertension
33.	D	Tracheal web
34.	B	Maxillary nerve (V2)
35.	D	Regular assessment of weight and height
36.	B	Steven-Johnson syndrome
37.	B	Tinnitus
38.	D	Pendred syndrome
39.	C	Palatine
40.	B	Recreates the antihelix by incorporating permanent scapha chonchal and scapha fossa triangularis horizontal mattress stitches
41.	C	Otosclerosis
42.	D	Relapsing polychondritis
43.	B	Glossopharyngeal nerve
44.	C	Churg Strauss
45.	B	Uses electrical frequency from 300kHz to 3 MHz
46.	B	Foreign body
47.	B	University of Pennsylvania Smell Identification Test
48.	C	The veins have no valves
49.	D C	4
50.	B	Is caused by constitutional activation of the G-protein
51.	C	Do you need any time off between 9-5pm during the week for religious purposes?

52.	C	Pott's puffy tumour
53.	E	Epstein Barr virus
54.	B	HPV 11
55.	D	Insert grommets
56.	D	Hormonal rhinitis
57.	E	Sixth branchial apparatus
58.	A	Foramen magnum
59.	B	Pterygopalatine fossa
60.	B	2cm
61.	D	T1
62.	B	Serum and urine osmolality
63.	D	IgE
64.	A	15cm
65.	D	Oesophageal candidiasis
66.	C	The treatment of early detected disease improves the cure rate in 75% of patients
67.	A	Olfactory nerve
68.	D	The marginal mandibular branch of the facial nerve may be damaged by dissection just superficial to the platysma muscle
69.	C	The petrotympanic fissure
70.	E	5mg
71.	C	Aspirin
72.	B	Level II
73.	A	Otomize
74.	E	Moebius syndrome
75.	B	Medullary thyroid carcinoma
76.	D	Rhabdomyosarcoma
77.	C	Adenotonsillectomy
78.	C	Hypertension

79.	B	Battle's sign
80.	C	T1N1aM0
81.	B	Submucous cleft
82.	E	Brainstem implant
83.	E	MRI T2 images
84.	D	Pyramidal process
85.	E	Haemangioma
86.	A	Venous malformation
87.	E	IV Cefotaxime
88.	D	6/0 prolene
89.	E	Cochlear implant
90.	C	Klebsiella rhinoscleromatis
91.	D	>50%
92.	B	Pleomorphic adenoma
93.	A	Acting as a topical anticholinergic and inhibiting mucosal glandular secretion of the nasal cavity
94.	A	Rough endoplasmic reticulum
95.	B	Inner ear conductive presbyacusis
96.	D	Platinum
97.	A	The inferior turbinate is one of the lamellae
98.	D	4
99.	E	Spatula misting
100.	C	Anti-histamines
101.	C	Haemophilia A
102.	C	Pure tone audiometry
103.	A	Uncuffed fenestrated
104.	C	Send sample for B2 transferrin analysis
105.	A	Gastro-oesophageal reflux disease
106.	A	Pearson correlation coefficient
107.	D	Nasolacrimal duct blockage

108.	C	Translabyrinthine approach without brainstem implant
109.	B	Streptococcal
110.	A	Anterior ethmoidal
111.	C	40-60 years
112.	C	Fluticasone fuorate

1. Which of the following are recognised features of Multiple Endocrine Neoplasia Type IIa?

    (a)   Parathyroid adenoma
    (b)   Parathyroid carcinoma
    (c)   Phaeochromocytoma
    (d)   Marfanoid habitus
    (e)   Medullary carcinoma

2. A 10-year-old boy presents with an Arnold Chiari Malformation and is noted to have nystagmus. What is the most likely type of nystagmus to be present?

    (a)   Upbeat
    (b)   Downbeat
    (c)   Vertical
    (d)   Pendular
    (e)   Bidirectional

3. Elevation of the soft palate is considered to be part of which phase in the physiology of swallowing?

    (a)   Oral
    (b)   Oral and pharyngeal
    (c)   Pharyngeal
    (d)   Oesophageal
    (e)   None of the above

4. A 45-year-old man presents with a 6months history of a neck lump. Examination reveals a nodule in the right thyroid lobe and a 2 cm level 4 lymph node. Ultrasound scan revealed a 1cm lesion in the thyroid gland and FNAC suggests papillary carcinoma. What is the most appropriate TNM stage?

   (a) T1N1bM0
   (b) T2N0M0
   (c) T2N1M0
   (d) T3N0M0
   (e) T3N1M0

5. Which one of the following statements is true regarding hypercalcaemia?

   (a) May be due to primary, secondary or tertiary hyperparathyroidism
   (b) Can be suppressed with steroids in patients with primary hyperparathyroidism
   (c) Is commonly associated with diarrhoea
   (d) Occurs in about 10% of patients with renal calculi
   (e) Is a feature of myeloma

6. The cochlea is a spiral shaped cavity in the bony labyrinth, how many turns is it comprised of?

   (a) 1
   (b) 1.5
   (c) 2
   (d) 2.5
   (e) 3

7. Which of the following is INCORRECT regarding UPSIT?

   (a) Commonly called scratch and sniff test
   (b) The maximum score is 40
   (c) Consists of 4 booklets
   (d) A score of 10-15 indicates a malingerer
   (e) The shelf life is 5 years

8. What is the amount of adrenaline contained in 1ml of 1:80,000 adrenaline solution?

   (a) 5mcg
   (b) 50mcg
   (c) 12.5mg
   (d) 12.5mcg
   (e) 125mcg

9. Antro-choanal polyp is a benign solitary lesion. From where does is commonly arise?

   (a) Ethmoidal sinus
   (b) Maxillary sinus
   (c) Frontal sinus
   (d) Sphenoidal sinus
   (e) Posterior choana

10. To assess whether serum calcium changes twelve hours, one day and three days following total thyroidectomy is affected by the rank of surgeons. What is the single most suitable statistical test?

    (a) two sample (unpaired) Students t-test
    (b) two way analysis of variance (ANOVA)
    (c) Wilcoxon matched pair test
    (d) One way analysis of variance
    (e) Mann-Whitney U Test

11. A 43-year-old man is referred from a psychiatric ward with a lamb bone stuck in cricopharyngeus. On examination he is unable to swallow his saliva and is drooling. The patient is unable to give informed consent. Which of the following statements is the most appropriate next step?

    (a) Make patient ward of court
    (b) Obtain consent from next of kin
    (c) Obtain consent from the patient
    (d) Surgery can proceed
    (e) Surgery cannot proceed

12. A 4-month-old with suspicion of hearing loss. What is the single most appropriate investigation?

    (a) Visual reinforcement audiometry
    (b) Auditory brainstem response
    (c) Pure tone audiometry
    (d) Otoacoustic emissions
    (e) Speech discrimination test

13. Chronic otitis media has a higher rate in which population group?

    (a)   Caucasians
    (b)   Indians
    (c)   Chinese
    (d)   Africans
    (e)   Eskimos

14. Which of the following statements on laryngeal anatomy is incorrect?

    (a)   The larynx may be divided into the supraglottis, glottis and subglottis
    (b)   Both surfaces of the epiglottis are components of the supraglottis
    (c)   The glottis is 1 cm below the free medial edge of the vocal cord
    (d)   The false vocal fold is considered part of the supraglottis
    (e)   The subglottis end at the lower border of the cricoid cartilage

15. What grading system is used for subglottic stenosis?

    (a)   Brodsky grading
    (b)   Myer and Cotton
    (c)   House Brackman
    (d)   APGAR
    (e)   Levine scale

16. A previously fit and well 32 years old man presents in A&E with acute development of concentric erythematous lesions in mouth, eyes and genital, with photophobia and fever. Which condition would you suspect?

    (a) Lupus
    (b) Behcet's disease
    (c) Steven's-Johnson Syndrome
    (d) Pemphigus
    (e) Pemphigoid

17. With regards the UK Guidelines in ENT practice for tonsillectomy and the selection criteria to consider surgery; what is the number of episodes/year of tonsillitis required for listing a patient for bilateral tonsillectomies?

    (a) 3 episodes
    (b) 4 episodes
    (c) 5 episodes
    (d) 6 episodes
    (e) 7 episodes

18. The oral cavity includes all of the following, except...

    (a) soft palate
    (b) anterior 2/3 tongue
    (c) hard palate
    (d) anterior tonsillar pillar
    (e) lips

19. The carotid body contains both chemoreceptors and baroreceptors. These are stimulated under certain circumstances to maintain homeostasis. Which one of the following anatomical regions of the brain is stimulated by neuronal transmission from the carotid body?

    (a) The basal ganglia
    (b) The cerebellum
    (c) The hypothalamus
    (d) The pineal gland
    (e) The posterior pituitary gland

20. A 16-year-old male with Treacher Collins syndrome and grade 3 microtia. What is the most appropriate biomaterial to fix a prosthetic ear on?

    (a) Teflon
    (b) Copper
    (c) Titanium
    (d) Platinum
    (e) Silastic

21. A 78-year-old woman presents with anosmia and ageusia following a severe cold. MR and CT scanning are reported as normal. What would you advise him?

    (a) Gargle saline
    (b) Do not immerse in water
    (c) Reduce salt in diet
    (d) Stop smoking
    (e) Note and adhere to the sell by dates on food

22. A 15-year-old girl with cystic fibrosis develops a chest infection. What is the most likely pathogen?

   (a) Streptococcus pneumonia
   (b) Klebsiella
   (c) Haemophilus influenza
   (d) Staphylococcus aureus
   (e) Pseudomonas aeruginosa

23. A 45-year-old male presents complaining of difficulty initiating sleep, excessive daytime somnolence and frequent nocturnal awakenings. Polysomnography shows no apnoeas/hypopnoeas. However, there are 5 movements of the flexors of his lower limb every hour. What is the most likely diagnosis?

   (a) Periodic limb movement disorder
   (b) Narcolepsy
   (c) Upper airways resistance syndrome
   (d) Central sleep apnoea
   (e) Idiopathic hypersomnolence

24. According to the European Positional Paper 2007, the diagnosis of rhinosinusitis depends on which factor(s):

   (a) Symptoms and signs
   (b) Severity
   (c) Duration
   (d) Quality of life measures
   (e) All of the above

25. A 3-year-old girl presents with bilateral conductive hearing loss, hypoplastic maxilla and syndactyl of the hands and feet. Which of the following is the most likely syndrome?

   (a) Alport syndrome
   (b) Apert syndrome
   (c) CHARGE syndrome
   (d) Cogan's syndrome
   (e) Crouzon syndrome

26. A 52-year-old man presents with a 1 month history of hoarse voice. He takes oral antacid therapy for indigestion and denies any dysphagia. What is the most likely diagnosis?

   (a) Hypothyroidism
   (b) Candidiasis of the larynx
   (c) Chronic laryngitis
   (d) Laryngeal papillomatosis
   (e) Squamous cell carcinoma of the larynx

27. A 25-year-old woman presents complaining of marked episodic frontal headache associated with phonophobia and nasal congestion but no rhinorrhoea or droopy eyes. Each episodes last for hours and takes her to bed. A 2 week course of antibiotic and nasal decongestants were ineffective. What is the most likely diagnosis?

   (a) Cluster headache
   (b) Tension headache
   (c) Common migraine
   (d) Acute sinusitis
   (e) Atypical facial pain

28. A 32-year-old man was seen in ITU for tracheostomy decannulation. He was previously intubated because of generalised weakness and respiratory distress. He was noted to have bilateral facial nerve palsies. Six weeks prior to his admission he had a flu-like illness. Which is the most likely cause for his facial nerve palsy?

    (a) Stroke
    (b) Myasthenia gravis
    (c) Multiple sclerosis
    (a) Cerebello-pontine angle tumour
    (b) Guillian-Barre

29. Which nerve is responsible for detecting noxious olfactory stimuli?

    (a) Greater superficial petrosal
    (b) Lesser petrosal
    (c) Deep petrosal
    (d) Olfactory nerve
    (e) Trigeminal

30. A patient has an abscess in the left cerebellar hemisphere with associated vertigo. What type of nystagmus would you expect to see?

    (a) Pendular
    (b) Bidirectional
    (c) Rotatory to the left
    (d) Vertical up-beating
    (e) Horizontal to the left

31. Suppurative labyrinthisis may occur when bacteria invade the otic capsule. Which of the following symptom complexes reflects invasion of the petrous apex?

    (a) Severe vertigo with profound SNHL
    (b) Facial nerve palsy with SHNL
    (c) Facial paraesthesias with retro-orbital pain
    (d) Suppurative otorrhoea and facial nerve palsy
    (e) Retro-orbital pain and sixth nerve palsy

32. A 21-year-old university student presents with bilateral enlargement of the parotid glands. What is the most likely cause?

    (a) Mumps
    (b) Staphylococcus aureus infection
    (c) Drugs
    (d) Stones
    (e) Pleomorphic adenomas

33. When the change in hearing levels is assessed after ossicular reconstruction, a 95 percent confidence interval aids in data interpretation because it

    (a) Gives the range of results consistent with the data
    (b) Estimates the accuracy of observed results
    (c) Adjusts for systematic error that may have occurred when results were measured
    (d) Defines the variability of observed data relative to the mean
    (e) Ensures-adequate statistical power

34. A 60 year old man presents with a cystic lesion on the anterior border of the sternocleidomastoid muscle. FNA reveals straw coloured fluid with squamous debris only. What is the most likely diagnosis?

    (a) Squamous cell carcinoma
    (b) Branchial cyst
    (c) Actinomyces
    (d) Tuberculosis
    (e) Reactive lymphadenopathy

35. What are the origins and insertions of the lateral pterygoid muscle?

    (a) Greater wing of sphenoid bone, lateral pterygoid plate, condyloid process of the mandible and TMJ capsule
    (b) Lesser wing of sphenoid bone, lateral pterygoid plate, condyloid process of the mandible and TMJ capsule
    (c) Greater wing of sphenoid bone, medial pterygoid plate, condyloid process of the mandible and TMJ capsule
    (d) Lesser wing of sphenoid bone, medial pterygoid plate, coronoid process of the mandible and TMJ capsule
    (e) Greater wing of sphenoid bone, lateral pterygoid plate, coronoid process of the mandible and TMJ capsule

36. Which muscle divides the submandibular gland into superficial and deep lobes?

    (a) Digastric muscle
    (b) Mylohyoid
    (c) Omohyoid
    (d) Thyrohyoid
    (e) Sternocleidomastoid

37. Which of the following is preserved during a Level IV cordectomy (according to the European Laryngeal Society Cordectomy classification)?

   (a) Vocalis muscle
   (b) Vocal ligament
   (c) Vocal cover
   (d) Thyroarythenoid muscle
   (e) Cricoarythenoid muscle

38. A 29-year-old man presents with a lesion associated with an anaerobic gram-negative bacterium that produces sulphur like granules. What is the most likely diagnosis?

   (a) Behcet's disease
   (b) Hairy leukoplakia
   (c) Actinomycosis
   (d) Oral candidiasis
   (e) Amyloidosis

39. Which of the following develops from the 2nd branchial arch?

   (a) Stapes footplate
   (b) Manubrium of the malleus
   (c) Head of the malleus
   (d) Otic capsule
   (e) Short process of incus

40. A 21-year-old male presents with a swollen tongue and lips, which settled with to C1 esterase inhibitor therapy. What is the most likely diagnosis?

    (a) Erythema multiforme
    (b) Pemphigoid
    (c) Pemphigus
    (d) Hereditary angio-oedema
    (e) Median Rhomboid glossitis

41. A 70 year old man had a neck reconstruction with a free radial forearm flap. The first post-operative night, the SHO raised concerns about the flap and on examination it was pale but the capillary refill time was normal. The neck was re-explored the same night and you find the arterial and venous anastomosis intact. Which is the most likely cause for the flap failure?

    (a) Primary tissue rejection
    (b) Secondary tissue rejection
    (c) Atherosclerotic deposits in the anastomosed arteries
    (d) Post operative arterial vasoconstriction.
    (e) Too much intravenous fluids

42. A 2-year-old girl presents with suspicion of a hearing loss. What is the single most appropriate investigation?

    (a) Visual reinforcement audiometry
    (b) Auditory brainstem response
    (c) Pure tone audiometry
    (d) Otoacoustic emissions
    (e) Speech discrimination test

43. A 75-year-old woman presents complaining of clouding vision in her left eye after developing a rash over her left forehead. She also mention a burning pain over her left forehead and her left eye. Examination reveals no ptosis or diplopia and the corneal reflex is intact. What is the most likely nerve to be involved?

    (a) Cervical sympathetic plexus
    (b) Ophthalmic nerve
    (c) Short sphenopalatine nerve
    (d) Greater auricular nerve
    (e) Facial nerve

44. The risk of post-adenoidectomy haemorrhage using suction diathermy is?

    (a) 0.5%
    (b) 1.0%
    (c) 2%
    (d) 3%
    (e) 4%

45. With regards to House-Brackmann grading system of facial nerve palsy, which grading suggests at least an inability to close eyes completely?

    (a) Grade I
    (b) Grade II
    (c) Grade III
    (d) Grade IV
    (e) Grade V

46. Otosclerosis is an autosomal dominant metabolic bone disease which affects the endochondral layer of the otic capsule. What clinical sign is it associated with?

    (a) Battle sign
    (b) Schwartz sign
    (c) Rising sun sign
    (d) Bird-beak sign
    (e) Hitselberger's sign

47. A 78-year-old female presents with epiphora following excision of a basal cell carcinoma from beneath her left eye. Examination shows tension and eversion of the lower eyelid. What is the most likely diagnosis?

    (a) Blepharitis
    (b) Canalicular stenosis
    (c) Conjunctival disease
    (d) Ectropion
    (e) Punctual stenosis

48. Which of the following does NOT constitute a common finding of transverse temporal bone fracture?

    (a) anacusis
    (b) vertigo
    (c) facial nerve palsy
    (d) involvement of the foramen spinosum
    (e) fracture of the stylomastoid foramen

49. A 40-year-old barmaid presents with a 4 month history of a right throat discomfort. Examination reveals an indurated firm lesion in the right tonsil measuring 2.5cm and a a single ipsilateral lymph node, more than 3 cm but not more than 6 cm in greatest dimension in level 2 of the neck. What is the TNM stage?

    (a)   T1N1
    (b)   T1N2
    (c)   T2N1
    (d)   T2N2A
    (e)   T2N2B

50. A 72-year-old woman presents with a constant, throbbing generalised headache that has been increasing in intensity over a four week period. She also notices pain on chewing over the last 7 days. Examination reveals a low grade pyrexia and a tender scalp as well as decreased visual acuity in her right eye. ESR is elevated but her CRP and temporal artery biopsy are reported as normal. What is the single most likely cause for her headache?

    (a)   Temperomandibular joint (TMJ) dysfunction
    (b)   Meningitis
    (c)   Migraine
    (d)   Giant cell arteritis
    (e)   Space occupying lesion (e.g. brain tumour)

51. The muco-ciliary pathway is an important clearance mechanism. In which of the following is it not affected?

    (a)   Kartagener's syndrome
    (b)   Cystic Fibrosis
    (c)   Young's syndrome
    (d)   Pendred's syndrome
    (e)   Cigarette smoking

52. A 20-year-old Down syndrome male presents with difficulty breathing. Suspicious of a foreign body, a rigid bronchoscopy is performed and the trachea is seen to collapse (with the patient breathing spontaneously) but no foreign body is found. Which of the following is the most likely congenital abnormality?

    (a) Cleft palate
    (b) Submucous cleft
    (c) Tracheal stenosis
    (d) Tracheal web
    (e) Tracheomalacia

53. The nurse on the paediatric ward calls you regarding a 8 year old boy who is bleeding on the ward post tonsillectomy. His pre-op weight was 30 kg. He is conscious, orientated and alert but slightly pale. His pulse is 150/min , BP 100/80mmHg, capillary refill time is 4 seconds. What is the minimum amount of blood that he could have lost to give this clinical picture?

    (a) 20mls
    (b) 100mls
    (c) 200mls
    (d) 250mls
    (e) 350mls

54. Which of the following conditions is not associated with tinnitus?

    (a) Dural arteriovenous fistula
    (b) Otosclerosis
    (c) Acoustic neuroma
    (d) Presbyacussis
    (e) Otitis media

55. What is the commonest cause of otitis externa?

    (a) Pseudomonas aeruginosa
    (b) Staphylococcus aureus
    (c) Proteus
    (d) Escherichia coli
    (e) Fungal

56. A patient presents with unilateral deafness and vertigo. CT scan shows 'ground glass' appearance of the temporal bone. What is the most likely diagnosis?

    (a) Cholesteatoma
    (b) Cholesterol granuloma
    (c) Fibrous dysplasia
    (d) otosclerosis
    (e) chondroma

57. The risk of persistent perforation following short-term grommet insertion is?

    (a) 1 - 3%
    (b) 4 - 6%
    (c) 7 - 10%
    (d) 11-13%
    (e) 14-17%

58. Which of the following can cause hypercalcaemia?

    (a) Peptic ulcers
    (b) Acute myeloid leukaemia
    (c) Paget's disease
    (d) Sarcoidosis
    (e) Osteomalacia

59. What disease is characterized by Mikulicz's cells and causes stenosis of the nose, larynx and tracheobronchial tree?

    (a)   leprosy
    (b)   syphilis
    (c)   rhinoscleroma
    (d)   rhinophyma
    (e)   Wegener's granulomatosis

60. You are the consultant sitting in the coffee room discussing a piece of equipment with a company rep. Your SHO is doing a tonsillectomy under the supervision of the SpR. There was a change in the order of the list and you suddenly realised that the patient was consented for grommets only. One tonsil is out and haemostasis is in progress. What should you do?

    (a)   Stop the procedure and send the patient back to the ward
    (b)   Speak to the parents
    (c)   Take over and complete the procedures
    (d)   Let the SHO continue to take out the other tonsil and insert the grommets
    (e)   Ask the SpR to take over.

61. What surgical instrument is used to dissect the tonsil from its muscular attachments?

    (a)   Boyle-Davis
    (b)   Freer's elevator
    (c)   Gwynne Evans dissector
    (d)   St Claire Curette
    (e)   Mollison's pillar retractor

62. A 14-year-old girl presents with epistaxis. Nasal examination reveals a smooth swollen red mass with contact bleeding. What is the single most likely cause for the nose bleed?

    (a) Rhinolith
    (b) Pyogenic granuloma
    (c) Juvenile angiofibroma
    (d) Malignant disease
    (e) Idiopathic

63. A 67-year-old male presents with bilateral high frequency sensorineural hearing loss. What is the most likely diagnosis?

    (a) Menieres disease
    (b) Waadenburg syndrome type I
    (c) Waardenburg syndrome type IV
    (d) Pendred syndrome
    (e) Presbyacusis

64. The development of Nasopharyngeal carcinoma (NPC) is associated with genetic, viral and environmental factors . In which areas of the world is NPCs endemic?

    (a) In Northern America
    (b) In Southern China
    (c) In the Inuit population
    (d) In Western Africa
    (e) In Western Europe

65. What imaging modality is best for maxilla fractures?

  (a) Facial XR
  (b) Orthopantomogram
  (c) Ultrasound
  (d) CT scan
  (e) MRI scan

66. What is the only cranial nerve that exits from the dorsal aspect of the brainstem?

  (a) Olfactory nerve
  (b) Audiovestibular nerve
  (c) Abducens nerve
  (d) Occulomotor nerve
  (e) Trochlear nerve

67. The most important aspect of analysing and interpreting medical data is?

  (a) Choosing the right statistical test for the right dataset
  (b) Recognising uncertainty and quantifying error rates
  (c) Avoiding the multiple p-value problem by using multivariate techniques
  (d) Reporting statistical power whenever a significant p-value is obtained
  (e) Reporting statistical power whenever a non-significant p-value is obtained

68. Which of the following are contraindications to skin prick allergy testing?

   (a)   Patient taking antihistamines
   (b)   Patient with severe eczema
   (c)   Patient with dermatographism
   (d)   Patient with severe anaphylaxis
   (e)   All of the above

69. Which of the following is most commonly associated with carotid artery blow-out?

   (a)   Previous Radiation therapy
   (b)   Patient over 70 years
   (c)   The MacFee incision
   (d)   Smoking
   (e)   Diabetes

70. Cavernous sinus thrombosis may result from sinusitis, dental abscesses or orbital cellulitis. What early signs and symptoms would you expect?

   (a)   Hyperaesthesia in ophthalmic & maxillary divisions of the trigeminal nerve
   (b)   Facial nerve palsy
   (c)   Proptosis
   (d)   Decreased GCS
   (e)   Hyposmia

71. Which is the most likely causative virus for Laryngeal papillomatosis?

   (a) Herpes zoster virus
   (b) Epstein Barr Virus
   (c) Parvovirus
   (d) Human papilloma virus
   (e) Herpes simplex virus

72. A 10 year old boy presents with hearing loss, headaches and a firm mass in the left posterior triangle of the neck. Fine needle aspiration cytology of the neck mass reveals poorly differentiated malignant cells. The most likely source of the primary lesion is?

   (a)   tonsil
   (b)   tongue base
   (c)   piriform fossa
   (d)   nasopharynx
   (e)   oral cavity

73. A 3-year-old boy presents with recurrent abscesses and inflammation which mimics acute suppurative thyroiditis. Which branchial pouch is most likely to be responsible?

   (a)   First branchial pouch
   (b)   Second branchial pouch
   (c)   Third branchial pouch
   (d)   Fourth branchial pouch
   (e)   Sixth branchial pouch

74. Which skull base foramen is the exit port of the spinal division of the accessory out of the cranium?

   (a) Foramen Magnum
   (b) Jugular foramen
   (c) Hypoglossal foramen
   (d) Petrotympanic fissure
   (e) Stylomastoid foramen

75. The halo or ring sign on CT scan is indicative of…

   (a) Congenital otosclerosis
   (b) Cochlear otosclerosis
   (c) Pagets disease
   (d) Oval otosclerosis
   (e) Round window otosclerosis

76. With regards measures of central tendency in statistics; which one of the following statements is true?

   (a) The mean is always a good measure of central tendency
   (b) The mode is the sum of all the variables divided by the number of variables
   (c) The is only one mode in any given distribution
   (d) The mode is the middle of the distribution
   (e) The mean, mode and median are equal in normal distributions

77. In the evaluation of patients with maxillary sinus carcinoma, Ohngren's line can be drawn between?

    (a) The lateral and medial vault of the maxillary sinus
    (b) The angle of the mandible and the medial canthus
    (c) The infraorbital foramen and the nasal spine
    (d) The maxillary tuberosity and the condyle of the mandible
    (e) The inferior turbinate and the lateral canthus

78. A 23-year-old woman presents with dermatographism complains of excessive sneezing and runny nose. What is the single most appropriate investigation?

    (a) c-ANCA
    (b) p-ANCA
    (c) PR3
    (d) RAST
    (e) ACE

79. Which segment of the facial nerve is damaged if lacrimation and stapedial reflex are preserved, but movement of the muscle of the face and taste to the anterior 2/3 of the tongue are absent?

    (a) Meatal
    (b) Labyrnthine
    (c) Tympanic
    (d) Mastoid
    (e) Extracranial

80. Which test is most specific for Wegener's granulomatosis?

    (a) p-ANCA
    (b) c-ANCA
    (c) PR3
    (d) ACE
    (e) ANA

81. You are performing a laser resection of a papilloma on the nasopharyngeal surface of the soft palate using a laryngeal mirror. The mirror gets heated up during the procedure and the patient develops a 1x2cm mucosal burn on the posterior pharyngeal wall. What is you management plan?

    (a) Give analgesia and observe
    (b) Give steroids and observe
    (c) Give antibiotics and observe
    (d) Resect injured mucosa and allow to granulate
    (e) Resect the affected area and graft

82. A 48-year-old male presents with numbness of the upper left medial incisor following transantral surgery on his pterygopalatine fossa. What is the most likely nerve to be involved?

    (a) Anterior superior alveolar nerve
    (b) Anterior palatine nerve
    (c) Short sphenopalatine nerve
    (d) Long palatine nerve
    (e) Long sphenopalatine nerve

83. A 35-year-old woman presents with increasing difficulty in swallowing over the previous 3 months. This become worse as a meal progressed, and has been associated with 1 stone of weight loss. She also complains of general tiredness and weakness. What is the most likely diagnosis?

    (a) Globus pharyngeus
    (b) Myasthenia gravis
    (c) Pharyngeal pouch
    (d) Stroke
    (e) Goitre

84. Following a road traffic accident, a patient was noted to have a conductive hearing loss with an air-bone gap of 60dB. What is the most likely cause?

    (a) Fracture of the long process of the Incus
    (b) Fracture of the malleus
    (c) Dislocation of the stapes footplate
    (d) Fracture of the the stapes supra-structure
    (e) Dislocation of the incudo-stapedial joint

85. Which of the following topical aural preparation contains clioquinol?

    (a) Otomize
    (b) Otosporin
    (c) Sofradex
    (d) Betnovate
    (e) Locorten-Vioform

86. At what age will a normal child be able to recognise his/her parent voice and turn his/her head towards noise?

    (a)   0-3months
    (b)   4-6months
    (c)   7-10months
    (d)   11-14months
    (e)   16-18months

87. Which salivary gland produces 80 percent of resting saliva?

    (a)   Parotid glands
    (b)   Submandibular glands
    (c)   Sublingual glands
    (d)   Minor salivary glands
    (e)   Equal volumes from parotid & submandibular glands

88. What volume of saline is needed to make 1:200,000 solution using 1ml of 1:1000 adrenaline?

    (a)   10mls
    (b)   20mls
    (c)   100mls
    (d)   200mls
    (e)   400mls

89. A 43 year old businessman, with a BMI of 37, presents with loud snoring. His wife also mentions apnoeic episodes. Overnight pulse oximetry shows oxygen desaturation dips of below 86 percent over a 7 hour sleep period on 220 occasions. He suffers with severe claustrophobia. Select the next best option from the list below?

    (a)   Refer for a mandibular splint
    (b)   Refer for a trial of nasal CPAP
    (c)   Refer for polysomnography
    (d)   List for UVPP
    (e)   Refer to dietician for weight reduction

90. Which of the following is the commonest side effect of oral steroid usage in ENT practice?

    (a)   peptic ulceration
    (b)   tendon rupture
    (c)   Insomnia
    (d)   Skin rash
    (e)   Weight gain

91. A 60 year old patient presents with a 3cm thyroid nodule. Her past medical history included laryngeal cancer treated with radiotherapy. Fine needle aspiration cytology confirms the presence of malignant cells. Which is the most likely histological form of cancer?

    (a)   Papillary carcinoma
    (b)   Follicular carcinoma
    (c)   Medullary carcinoma
    (d)   Anaplastic carcinoma
    (e)   Lymphoma

92. What is the chemical constituent in Rinatec?

    (a) Iodoform, benzoin & storax
    (b) Iodoform Paraffin Bismuth
    (c) Fluticasone fuorate
    (d) Fluticasone proprionate
    (e) Ipratropium bromide

93. A 12 year old girl presents with a rapidly growing lesion on the soft palate without any lymphadenopathy. The most likely diagnosis is?

    (a) Pleomorphic adenoma
    (b) Adenoid cystic carcinoma
    (c) Accinic cell carcinoma
    (d) Mucoepidermoid carcinoma
    (e) Lymphoma

94. A 35-year-old male presents with excessive day time somnolence. Polysomnography shows no apnoeic episodes and 2 hypopnoeic episodes per hour. However, there are frequent snoring related arousals. Oesophageal manometry during sleep shows progressive increase in oesophageal pressure terminating in arousal. What is the most likely diagnosis?

    (a) Periodic limb movement disorder
    (b) Narcolepsy
    (c) Upper airways resistance syndrome
    (d) Central sleep apnoea
    (e) Idiopathic hypersomnolence

95. What grading system is used for pars tensa retraction pockets?

    (a) Tos
    (b) Sadé
    (c) Chandlers
    (d) House-Brackman
    (e) Brighton grading

96. A 34-year-old male diver presents with nausea and vertigo on hearing a loud noise. What is the most likely diagnosis?

    (a) Boyce's sign
    (b) Tullio phenomena
    (c) Alexander's law
    (d) Arnold's reflex
    (e) Grisel sign

97. With regards Bone Anchored Hearing aids, which of the following statements is not true?

    (a) Should only be used if the bone conduction hearing is better than 45 dB
    (b) The screw is made of titanium
    (c) Can be used for bilateral canal atresia
    (d) Can be used for single sided deafness
    (e) Is placed on the mastoid bone most frequently

98. Which of the following mechanism provides the maximum impedance matching in the middle ear?

    (a) Lever effect of the ossicular chain
    (b) Baffle effect of the tympanic membrane, i.e., phase difference between conduction at oval window and round window
    (c) Size of the ear canal
    (d) Area effect of the tympanic membrane relative to the stapes foot plate
    (e) Size and direction of the pinna

99. A 5month old British born child is referred because of parental concerns about his hearing. Which investigation do you organize?

    (a) Otoacoustic emmissions
    (b) Electrocochleography
    (c) Auditory brainstem response
    (d) Cortical evoked response audiometry
    (e) Distraction test

100. A 16-year-old boy presents with severe left-sided maxillary sinusitis following a upper respiratory tract infection. What is the most likely pathogen?

    (a) Streptococcus pneumonia
    (b) Streptococcus milleri
    (c) Haemophilus influenza
    (d) Staphylococcus aureus
    (e) Pseudomonas aeruginosa

101. A 65 year old patient had a total laryngectomy and comprehensive neck dissection for a T4N2bM0 hypopharyngeal carcinoma. Two months after post-operative radiotherapy, he developed a pharyngocutaneous fistula. What is the best course of action?

   (a)   EUA and biopsy
   (b)   MRI
   (c)   CT
   (d)   Close with a flap
   (e)   Wait and watch

102. A 55-year patient has persistent symptoms from a possible foreign body in the oro-hypopharynx. What would be the next appropriate investigation?

   (a)   Reassure and discharge
   (b)   Ultrasound neck
   (c)   CT scan
   (d)   MRI
   (e)   Surgical intervention

103. Patients with Down syndrome are prone to recurrent episodes of croup. This is most likely due to...

   (a)   Recurrent tonsillitis with tonsillar hypertrophy
   (b)   Depressed immunity
   (c)   macroglossia
   (d)   high incidence of OSA
   (e)   subglottic narrowing

104. Cholesteatoma consists of layers of keratin lined by which type of epithelium?

    (a)   Squamous epithelium
    (b)   Simple cuboidal epithelium
    (c)   Simple columnar epithelium
    (d)   Ciliated columnar epithelium
    (e)   Glandular epithelium

105. A 36-year-old overweight woman presents with episodic vertigo, hearing loss, tinnitus and fullness in her right ear. What would you advise him?

    (a)   Lose weight
    (b)   Reduce salt in diet
    (c)   Note and adhere to the sell by dates on food
    (d)   Gargle saline
    (e)   Place icepacks on forehead

106. A 14-year-old boy presents with fever, arthralgia and facial nerve palsy following an adventure holiday in Sweden. What is the most likely infective organism?

    (a)   Borellia burgdorferi
    (b)   Atypical mycobacterium
    (c)   Actinomyces
    (d)   Rochalimaea (Bartonella) henselae
    (e)   Rhinosporidium seeberi

107. A cystic lesion without a true epithelial lining. What is the most likely corresponding lesion?

  (a) Lymphangioma
  (b) Salivary mucocele
  (c) Ranula
  (d) Adenoid cystic carcinoma
  (e) Mucoepidermoid carcinoma

108. A 40-year-old male air traffic controller complains of severe nasal blockage and rhinorrhoea when out working in the cold. His symptoms persist to a lesser degree when not working. What is the most likely diagnosis?

  (a) Atrophic rhinitis
  (b) Allergic rhinitis
  (c) Drug induced rhinitis
  (d) Hormonal rhinitis
  (e) Non allergic occupational rhinitis

109. Transplant between identical twins is known as...

  (a) Allograft
  (b) Homograft
  (c) Autograft
  (d) Isograft
  (e) Xenograft

110. A 10-year-old boy presents with progressive sensorineural hearing loss, which suddenly worsens following head trauma whilst playing rugby. What is the single most likely diagnosis?

    (a)   Hereditodegenerative disease of the cochlea
    (b)   Ushers syndrome
    (c)   Cochlear hydrops
    (d)   Enlarged vestibular aqueduct syndrome
    (e)   Cogan's syndrome

111. A patient presents with a short history of acute sinusitis, marked pyrexia, bilateral chemosis and 3rd nerve palsy. What is the most likely diagnosis?

    (a)   Periorbital cellulitis
    (b)   Gradenigo's syndrome
    (c)   Cavernous sinus thrombosis
    (d)   A brain abscess
    (e)   An orbital abscess

112. Which of the following are sensori-neural causes for anosmia?

    (a)   Rhinitis
    (b)   Nasal polyps
    (c)   Encephalocoeles
    (d)   Dermoid cysts
    (e)   Sarcoidosis

		PAPER SIX
		Answers
1.	D	Marfanoid habitus
2.	B	Downbeat
3.	C	Pharyngeal
4.	C	T2N1M0
5.	E	Is a feature of myeloma
6.	D	2.5
7.	D	A score of 10-15 indicates a malingerer
8.	D	12.5mcg
9.	B	Maxillary sinus
10.	B	Two way analysis of variance (ANOVA)
11.	D	Surgery can proceed
12.	D	Otoacoustic emissions
13.	E	Eskimos
14.	C	The glottis is 1 cm below the free medial edge of the vocal cord
15.	B	Myer & Cotton
16.	C	Stevens-Johnson syndrome
17.	E	7 episodes
18.	A	Soft palate
19.	C	The hypothalamus
20.	C	Titanium
21.	E	Note & adhere to the sell by date on foods
22.	E	Pseudomonas aeruginosa
23.	A	Periodic limb movement disorder
24.	E	All of the above
25.	B	Apert syndrome
26.	C	Chronic laryngitis
27.	C	Common migraine
28.	B	Guillian Barre

29.	E	Trigeminal
30.	E	Horizontal to the left
31.	E	Retro-orbital pain & sixth nerve palsy
32.	A	Mumps
33.	D	Defines the variability of observed data relative to the mean
34.	A	Squamous cell carcinoma
35.	A	Greater wing of sphenoid bone, lateral pterygoid plate, condyloid process of the mandible and TMJ capsule
36.	B	Mylohyoid
37.	C	Cricoarythenoid muscle
38.	C	Actinomycosis
39.	B	Manubrium of the malleus
40.	D	Hereditary angio-oedema
41.	D	Post operative arterial vasoconstriction.
42.	A	Visual reinforcement audiometry
43.	B	Ophthalmic nerve
44.	A	0.5%
45.	D	Grade IV
46.	B	Schwartz sign
47.	D	Ectropion
48.	E	Fracture of the stylomastoid foramen
49.	D	T2N2A
50.	D	Giant cell arteritis
51.	D	Pendred syndrome
52.	E	Tracheomalacia
53.	D	250mls
54.	B	Otosclerosis
55.	A	Pseudomonas aeruginosa
56.	C	Fibrous dysplasia

57.	A	1-3%
58.	D	Sarcoidosis
59.	C	Rhinoscleroma
60.	B	Speak to the parents
61.	C	Gwynne Evans dissector
62.	B	Pyogenic granuloma
63.	E	Presbyacusis
64.	B	Southern China
65.	D	CT Scan
66.	E	Trochlear nerve
67.	B	Recognising uncertainty and quantifying error rates
68.	E	All of the above
69.	A	Previous radiation therpy
70.	C	Proptosis
71.	D	Human papilloma virus
72.	D	Nasopharynx
73.	C	Third branchial pouch
74.	B	Jugular foramen
75.	B	Cochlear otosclerosis
76.	E	The mean, mode and median are equal in normal distributions
77.	B	The angle of the mandible and the medial canthus
78.	D	RAST
79.	D	Mastoid
80.	B	c-ANCA
81.	A	Give analgesia and observe
82.	A	Anterior superior alveolar nerve
83.	B	Myasthenia gravis
84.	E	Dislocation of the incudo-stapedial joint

85.	E	Locorten-Vioform *(also Betnovate-C)*
86.	B	4-6months
87.	B	Submandibular glands
88.	D	200mls
89.	A	Refer for a mandibular splint
90.	C	Insomnia
91.	A	Papillary carcinoma
92.	E	Ipratropium bromide
93.	D	Mucoepidermoid carcinoma
94.	C	Upper airways resistance syndrome
95.	B	Sade
96.	B	Tullio phenomena
97.	E	Is placed on the mastoid bone most frequently
98.	D	Area effect of the tympanic membrane relative to the stapes foot plate
99.	C	Auditory brainstem response
100.	A	Streptococcus pneumonia
101.	A	EUA & biopsy
102.	C	CT Scan
103.	E	Subglottic narrowing
104.	A	Squamous epithelium
105.	B	Reduce salt in diet
106.	A	Borellia burgdorferi
107.	B	Salivary mucocele
108.	E	Non allergic occupational rhinitis
109.	D	Isograft
110.	D	Enlarged vestibular aqueduct syndrome
111.	C	Cavernous sinus thrombosis
112.	E	Sarcoidosis

Reprint of #895775 - C0 - 197/132/17 - PB - Lamination Gloss - Printed on 26-Mar-19 12:03